MAMMOGRAPHY TECHNIQUES AND REVIEW

Edited by **Fabiano Cavalcanti Fernandes,**
Lourdes Mattos Brasil
and **Renato da Veiga Guadagnin**

Mammography Techniques and Review
http://dx.doi.org/10.5772/58670
Edited by Fabiano Cavalcanti Fernandes, Lourdes Mattos Brasil and Renato da Veiga Guadagnin

Contributors
Mónica Vieira Martins, Michal Haindl, Vaclav Remes, Alexander Karpov, Serban Nastasia, Cleber Da Silva Alves, Lourdes Brasil, Marilia Miranda Forte Gomes, Fátima Elpidio

Published by InTech
Janeza Trdine 9, 51000 Rijeka, Croatia

Publishing Process Manager Iva Lipovic
Technical Editor InTech DTP team
Cover InTech Design team

First published June, 2015
Printed in Croatia

Additional hard copies can be obtained from orders@intechopen.com

Mammography Techniques and Review, Edited by Fabiano Cavalcanti Fernandes, Lourdes Mattos Brasil and Renato da Veiga Guadagnin
p. cm.
ISBN 978-953-51-2138-1

For EU product safety concerns:
IN TECH d.o.o., Prolaz Marije Krucifikse Kozulić 3, 51000 Rijeka, Croatia,
info@intechopen.com or visit our website at intechopen.com.

Meet the editors

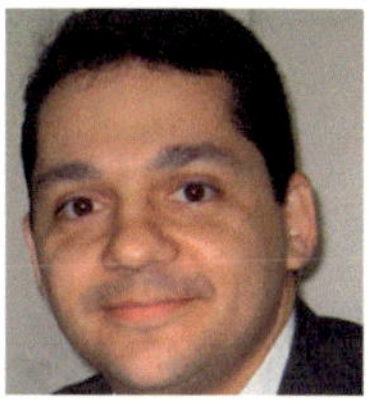

Fabiano Cavalcanti Fernandes, PD. in Computer Science, Federal University of Paraiba (1998), Master of Science in Knowledge Management and Technology Information, Catholic University of Brasilia (2007), Doctorate in Biotechnology (Bioinformatics), Catholic University of Brasilia (2012). He is currently professor at Federal Institute of Brasilia. His scientific works concern bioinformatics, artificial intelligence, data mining, data science, machine learning and informatics in health.

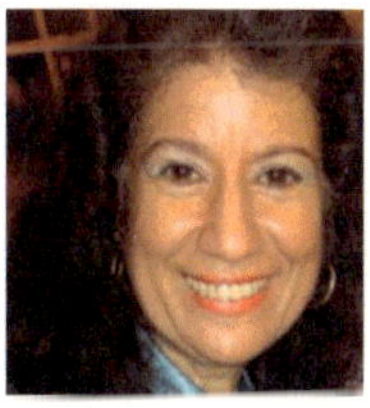

Lourdes Mattos Brasil, PhD Electrical Engineer, Federal University of Santa Catarina (1984), Master of Science in Electrical Engineering/Biomedical Engineering, Federal University of Santa Catarina (1994), Sandwich Doctorate in Mathematical Applied from Facultes Universitaires Notre_Dame de La Paix (FUNDP), Belgium (1997–1998) and D.Sc. in Electrical Engineering/Biomedical Engineering (1999). She is currently professor/researcher/head of the Lato Sensu in Clinical Engineering Course and Post-Graduation Program in Biomedical Engineering, besides being professor of the Course of Electronic Engineering, at the University of Brasilia at Gama, Brazil. Her scientific works concern artificial intelligence, data mining, machine learning, knowledge acquisition, knowledge based systems, hybrid expert systems, virtual reality, intelligent tutoring systems, informatics in health, e–learning and nanotechnology.

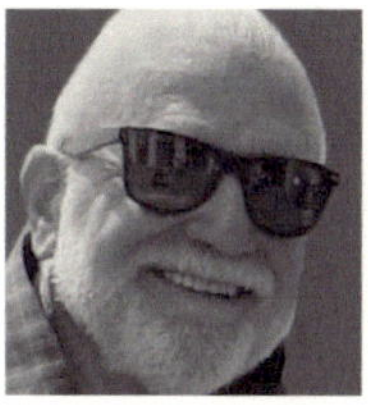

Renato da Veiga Guadagnin, Dr. rer. publ. Mechanical Engineer at Polytechnic School in Federal University of Rio de Janeiro (1969), MS course on Systems Analysis at the National Institute for Space Research, in São José dos Campos (1972) and Ph.D studies at the German University of Administrative Sciences Speyer, Germany (1983). He is a retired professor from the University of Brasilia. He is currently adjunct professor at Catholic University of Brasilia. He has academic and management experience in Computer Science, with research interests in applications on automatic image modeling and analysis in health areas, knowledge visualization, artificial intelligence to support decision making.

Contents

Preface

Mammography remains at the backbone of medical tools to examine the human breast. The early detection of breast cancer typically uses adjunct tests to mammogram such as ultrasound, positron emission mammography, electrical impedance, Computer-aided detection systems and others. In the present digital era it is even more important to use the best new techniques and systems available to improve the correct diagnosis and to prevent mortality from breast cancer.

This book is designed to provide an up to date impression of the state-of-the-art in mammography techniques and new trends. Each chapter contains a review or future directions and challenges in their respective areas. I hope the reader can obtain an accurate impression of the pace of research in these areas. Nevertheless, the breast cancer detection exams continually present new challenges. Will the new techniques and methods ever be able to prevent breast cancer before it indeed occurs? Will the new methods combined with Computer-aided Artificial Intelligence Systems withdraw the physicians from the process? That questions remains uncertain, but clearly the field will remain an exciting research area for many years to come.

Fabiano Cavalcanti Fernandes
Federal Institute of Brasilia (IFB), Brazil

Lourdes Mattos Brasil
University of Brasilia (UnB), Brazil

Renato da Veiga Guadagnin
Catholic University of Brasilia (UCB), Brazil

Chapter 1

An Electrical Impedance Mammographic Scheme — Norms and Pathology

Alexander Karpov, Andrey Kolobanov and
Marina Korotkova

Additional information is available at the end of the chapter

http://dx.doi.org/10.5772/60014

1. Introduction

1.1. The concept of a normal mammographic scheme: mammographic schemes in diagnostics

A normal mammographic scheme in traditional diagnostic techniques (X-ray, US) is a set of anatomic structures regularly found on normal mammograms. Existing classifications of normal breast X-ray anatomic pictures help distinguish several structural types of the breast. Each structural type is presented by a certain morphological substrate (Figure 1). Wolfe's Classification (1976),

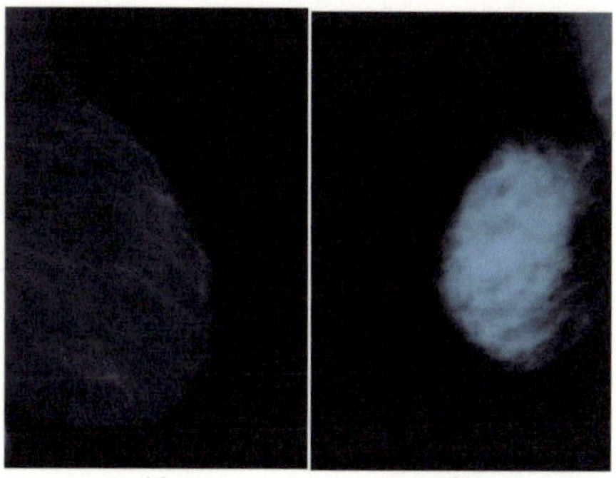

Figure 1. (a) Predominantly fatty normal mammogram; (b) dense normal mammogram.

Tabar's Classification (1997), Boyd's Classification (1980) and the BI-RADS Classification (2000) are the most widely-known [1, 2, 3]. According to Wolfe, breast structural types are defined by the ratio of fat to ducts: N1 – the breast consists mainly of fat; P1 – linear densities occupy no more than 25% of the breast; P2 – linear densities occupy more than 25% of the breast; Dy – dense. Tabar relies on histomammographic correlations and distinguishes five types of breast structure: I – a balanced proportion of all components of the breast tissue; II – fat breasts; III – a predominance of fat tissue with retroareolar residual fibrous tissue; IV – predominantly nodular densities; V – dense breasts. Boyd takes a different approach, introducing a quantitative evaluation of the breast structure: A – 0% mammographic density; B - >0-10%; C - >10-25%; D - >25-50%; E - >50-75%; F - >75%. The BI-RADS classification modifies that worked out by Wolfe, expressing a breast density percentage and adding a division into quartiles: Type 1 – extremely fat, with parenchyma below 25%; Type 2- minimal density, parenchyma 25-50%; Type 3 – heterogeneous density, parenchyma 50-75%; Type 4 – extremely dense, parenchyma 75-100%. Thus, breast structural types have been defined in reliance on the correlation between the ductal component and fat lobules. The breast has a variable appearance in each case and the breast density decreases after the menopause. It should be noted that no similar system of breast structural types has been developed by reference to the US.

A distortion of the normal mammographic scheme is observed when structural changes appear, in the form of pathological shadows and microcalcinations. Such focal changes are easily detected by medical devices diagnosing using tissue density. However, focal changes are not the only mode of cancer manifestation. Diffuse changes of the breast structure may also stand for a malignant process and may equally result in the distortion of the mammographic scheme. Diffuse changes do not affect breast tissue density and present certain difficulties for X-ray diagnostics.

2. Electrical impedance images

Electrical impedance mammography is a medical imaging technique aimed at creating images of the breast by means of external scanning. Electrical impedance mammography measures electromagnetic phenomena and belongs to non-invasive techniques of image creation [4].

There exist two types of techniques creating tomographic images: local and non-local. X-ray computer tomography, magnetic resonance tomography and positron emission tomography belong to local techniques, implying the passage of one direct ray through the body and the creation of one pixel in the image (one ray – one pixel). The pixel value depends solely on the substance that the ray meets on its way. Using multiple angles for calculation captures two-dimensional slices that can be reconstructed for obtaining three-dimensional images of the object scanned.

Electrical impedance mammography belongs to the category of soft-field tomography and uses a non-local technique for image creation, whereby all points on the object scanned affect the measurement result. This is why the value of the mean electrical conductivity is dominant in detecting focal changes.

We use the electrical impedance computer mammographer MEIK 5.6 for the creation of electrical impedance images [5, 6]. The mammographer has the following key characteristics:

- Electrode configuration. A planar set of electrodes is used for the procedure. Electrodes configured in this way have a coplanar location. In our case, the electrodes are arranged on the platform of the mammographer, which is pressed to the breast and immobilized manually. The advantages of using electrodes with a planar configuration include the following. First, the electrodes are fixed onto the panel so that their position is exact. This allows the avoidance of any positional error. Second, the scanning panel is handy and manoeuvrable, so it can be easily moved along the patient's body. This means that the device is designed for real-time use. Third, the sensitivity of the linear electrodes is relatively more concentrated than that of the electrodes surrounding the area of interest in the form of a circle, which is why the resolution may increase locally.

- Data collection method. When carrying out an electrical impedance examination, a set of electrodes is placed on the object's surface. A part of each electrode is used as an inductor, the other part as a measuring electrode. An electrical supply is generally used as an inductor, while the difference in the electric potential is measured between the measuring electrodes. All the measurements are done on the object's surface. The main goal is to reconstruct the volumetric distribution of the object's conductivity with the results of the electric measurements on its surface.

- Image reconstruction algorithm. A back-projection algorithm is used for the reconstruction of a volumetric static frequency image along the equipotential surfaces of the electric field with the weight function applied both horizontally and vertically. The image is reconstructed in layers that are located parallel to the panel with the electrodes. The back-projection method was originally worked out as an empirical method. It was based on the idea of the direct distribution of scanning radiation in the tissue (i.e., the presence of rays). Electrical impedance mammography is not based on the use of rays, which leads us to introduce the term 'pseudoray'. The use of this term is justified by the fact that the change in the superficial difference of electric potential (as compared to homogeneous tissues) invoked by the presence in the object of a local non-homogeneous area is generally concentrated in the segment that is a projection of the non-homogeneity onto the object's surface along the equipotential lines (or surfaces) of the field.

Thus, the method of back-projection may be applied to the case when the power lines of electric field intensity are used instead of rays, the former being estimated for the case of homogeneous conductivity distribution [7].

A two-dimensional image is a good way to illustrate the method. The figure on the left (Figure 2) shows systems of equipotential lines for two injecting electrodes *i(A)иi(B)*.

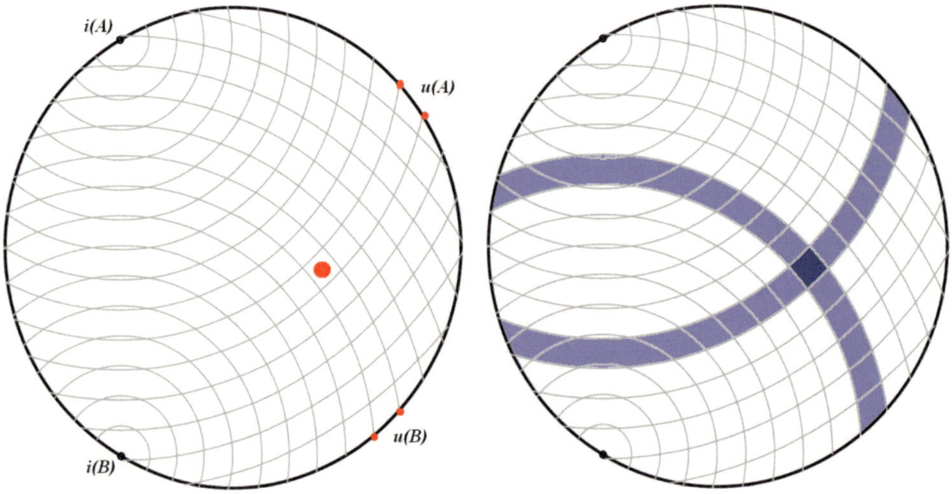

Figure 2. Equipotential lines – pseudorays and image reconstruction.

Here, we present the case of a diametrical location of an injection electrode pair (the opposing referent electrode is not shown in the figure). The red spot stands for a non-homogeneous area in the object. The red dots on the surface of the object show pairs of measuring electrodes in which the electric potential differences u(A) and u(B) diverge maximally as compared to areas with a homogeneous distribution of electrical conductivity. The figure on the right demonstrates the principle of image reconstruction based on measurement results obtained from two injecting electrodes. The light blue lines show the noise components of the reconstructed image. The dark blue cross-section is a constructed image of the non-homogeneous area. The image will be of better quality when reconstructed by measurement results from a greater number of injecting electrodes.

The key differences between the three-dimensional image and the two-dimensional image involve the following:

- Equipotential surfaces have a spherical shape with a centre in the injecting electrode;
- The projection of an isolated non-homogeneity along the equipotential lines onto the object's surface has a spherical shape with a centre in the injecting electrode and a radius equal to the distance from the injecting electrode to the non-homogeneity;
- The change in the superficial potential differences (as compared to the homogeneous tissues) is generally concentrated in the circle shown above, and decreases as the distance between the point in the circle and the non-homogeneity becomes greater.

Thus, the back-projection method in a three-dimensional image consists of the usual projection of the superficial potential difference change (as compared to the homogeneous tissues) into the object along the equipotential surfaces, but with a weight depending on the distance between the projected point and the point at which conductivity reconstruction occurs [7].

3. Elements of electrical impedance in a mammographic scheme

Here, we present a description of breast anatomic structures and comment on the concept of a mammographic scheme in terms of electrical impedance mammography [8].

3.1. Terminology

- Electrical conductivity scale - electrical conductivity index values from 0 to 1.00; or in grey-scale - changes from black to white, respectively.
- Hyperimpedance structure, lesion – the electrical conductivity is lower than the electrical conductivity of the surrounding tissue of the breast and corresponds to IC < 0.20.
- Isoimpedance structure, lesion – the electrical conductivity is approximately equal to the electrical conductivity of the surrounding tissue of the breast and corresponds to IC = 0.30-0.50 (this depends on the value of the mean electric conductivity).
- Hypoimpedance structure, lesion – the electrical conductivity is higher than the electrical conductivity of the surrounding tissue of the breast and corresponds to IC = 0.60-0.80 (this depends on the value of the mean electric conductivity).
- Animpedance structure, lesion – the electrical conductivity is considerably higher than the electrical conductivity of the surrounding tissue of the breast and corresponds to IC > 0.80 (this depends on the value of the mean electric conductivity).
- IC – index conductivity.

In the anatomy of the mammary gland, the following elements of the electrical mammographic scheme can be marked out: capsule, connective tissue carcass, parenchyma, secretory reservoir, nipple and areola.

3.2. Capsule

The mammary gland capsule consists of leaves of the superficial fascia and subcutaneous fat enveloping the mammary gland on all sides.

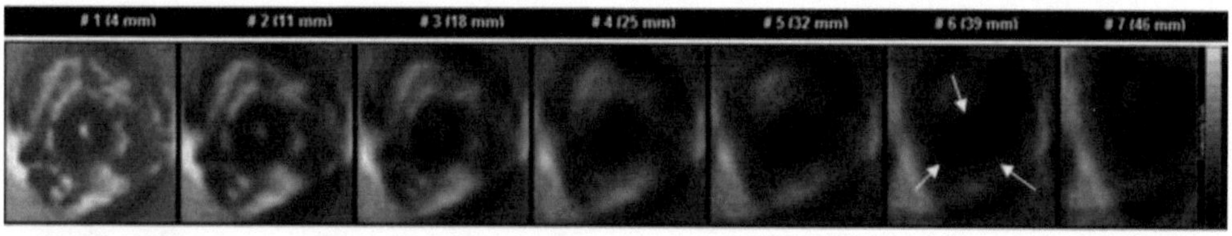

Figure 3. Electrical impedance tomogram of the mammary gland (EIM). Seven planes of scanning. In the sixth and the seventh scans, a retromammary tissue is visualized.

In the image, the capsule forms an important element of the mammographic scheme – the mammary gland contour – with fatty tissue intimately embracing the body of the mammary gland (capsulaadiposamammae). The front layer of the capsule ends in the behind-areola area where the ends of the milk duct are situated. In figure 3, one can see an electrical impedance tomogram where fatty tissue on the periphery of the mammary gland is represented in the shape of a hyperimpedance contour.

3.3. Carcass

The mammary gland is enclosed in a connective tissue capsule, sending septa into the strata of the gland. The septa consist of tender fibrillary tissues and are situated between the glandular elements. The septa that form the connective tissue framework of the mammary gland are in hyperimpedance and radically diverge from the areola. On the periphery of the mammary gland, the adipose capsule stands out in the form of a hyperimpedance contour (Figure 4).

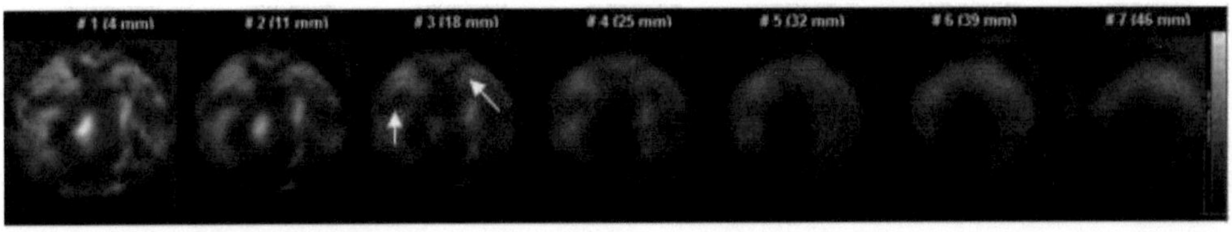

Figure 4. EIM. Seven planes of scan. In the first, second and third scans, the connective tissues' septa are visualized along with the radially diverging areolae.

3.4. Parenchyma

The parenchyma is a structural component of the mammary gland made of alveotubular glands and the connective tissue stroma. Alveotubular glands consisting of ductal and secretary epithelium are gathered into small lobules forming lobes. The connective tissue stroma is represented by a small number of cells, gentle tissues and the base material. Figure 5 shows an electrical impedance tomogram, where the parenchyma is represented in the form of isoimpedance areas visible between the septa.

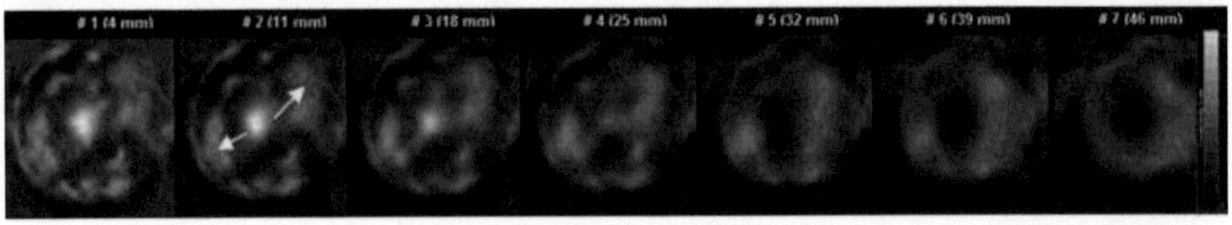

Figure 5. EIM. Seven scan planes. The parenchyma is visualized in the form of isoimpedance areas between the connective tissue septa.

3.5. Secretory reservoir

Before opening into the nipple milk ducts enlarge and form a lactiferous sinus (sinus lactiferi). It which accumulates secretion or milk produced in alveoli and is characterized by low electrical impedance. There are 15-25 such sinuses in the area behind the nipple. In Figure 6, one can see an electrical impedance tomogram where the lactiferous sinus zone visualizes itself as a vast hypoimpedance area, situated in the centre of the mammogram.

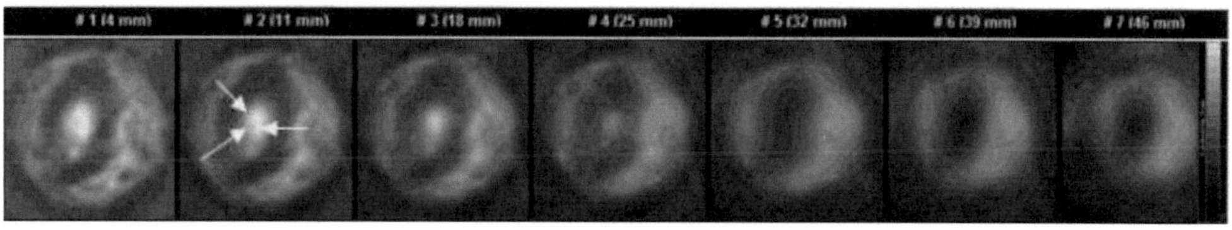

Figure 6. EIM. Seven scan planes. In the centre of the tomogram there is a hypoimpedance area corresponding to the location of the lactiferous sinuses.

3.6. Nipple and areola

The nipple of the mammary gland and the mammary areola are areas of hairless pigmented epidermis. The nipple consists of the lactiferous sinus, an extension into which flows the excretory ducts of the mammary gland lobules, with fibrous tissue around them, and a large number of sebaceous glands. The absence in the nipple of the perspiratory gland's excretory ducts defines its high electrical impedance. The nipple is visible in the first and second scans of the electrical impedance tomogram, taking the form of a linear hyperimpedance formation located in the centre, near the zone of the lactiferous sinuses (Figure 7).

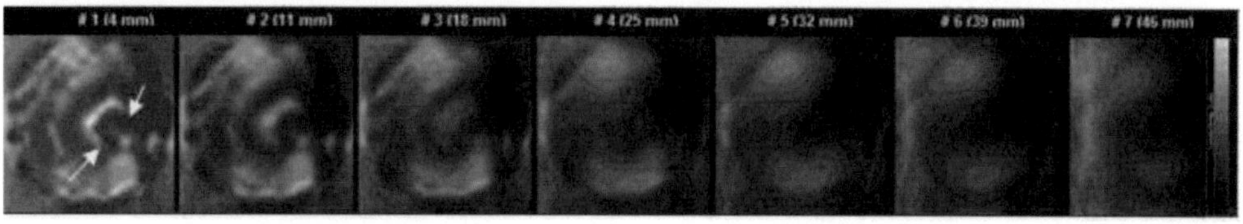

Figure 7. EIM. Seven scan planes. Outer segment. In the center of the 1st and the 2nd scans a linear hyperimpedance formation typical of the nipple is visualized.

The derma of the mammary areola contains a large number of pigmentary cells which condition its high electrical impedance. On the electrical impedance tomogram, the mammary areola is visualized as a hyperimpedance formation of a round shape around the area of the lactiferous sinuses (Figure 8).

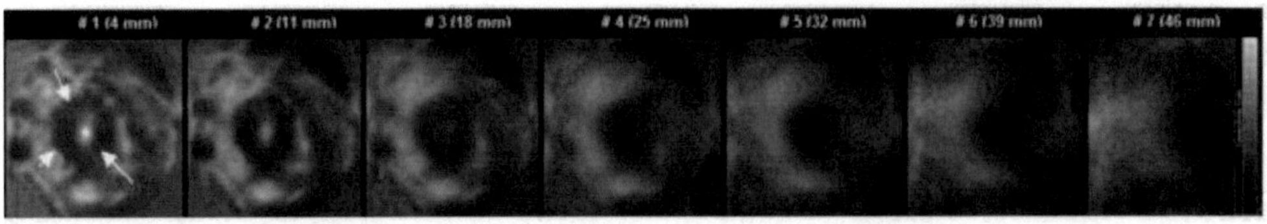

Figure 8. Impedance area in the centre of the tomogram corresponding to the placement of the areola.

4. Normal electrical impedance mammographic scheme

As has been mentioned above, the breast may have a variable appearance on the tomogram. This is why the electrical impedance mammographic scheme depends on the type of breast structure. Earlier, we pointed out five types of breast structure from the point of view of electrical impedance mammography execution (Table 1).

	EIM classification	*ACR classification*
Type Ia	Amorphous type of mammary gland structure. IC = above 0.66 *IC – index conductivity	Predominantly fat. Under 25% of the tissue is represented by the parenchyma.
Type Ib	Mixed type of mammary gland structure with amorphous component predominance. IC=0.57-0.65.	
Type II	Mixed type of mammary gland structure. IC=0.30-0.56	Fat with some fibroglandular tissue. 25-50% of the tissue is represented by the parenchyma.
Type III	Mixed type of mammary gland structure with an acinal/ductal component predominance. High density of the acinal/ductal component. IC=0.22-0.29.	Heterogeneously dense. 50-75% of the tissue is represented by the parenchyma.
Type IV	Acinal/ductal type of mammary gland structure. Extremely high density of the acinal/duct component. IC <0.22.	Extremely dense. 75-100% of the parenchyma tissue.

Table 1. Mammary gland structure from the perspective of electrical impedance mammography execution, and breast density types according to the classification of the American College of Radiology (ACR).

4.1. Normal mammographic scheme with a ductal-type mammary gland structure

The prevailing ductal component in the parenchyma structure is typical of women during the early reproductive period. The high density of the ductal component is a significant obstacle in the way of electric charges, which adds specific features to the electrical impedance image: the prevalence of darker tones of greyscale; well-defined anatomical landmarks; low values of electrical conductivity. In the normal electrical impedance mammographic scheme, the anatomical landmarks are distinct and well-defined.

- The mammary gland contour is even and regular, without extrusions, retractions or unilateral thickening (Figure 9).

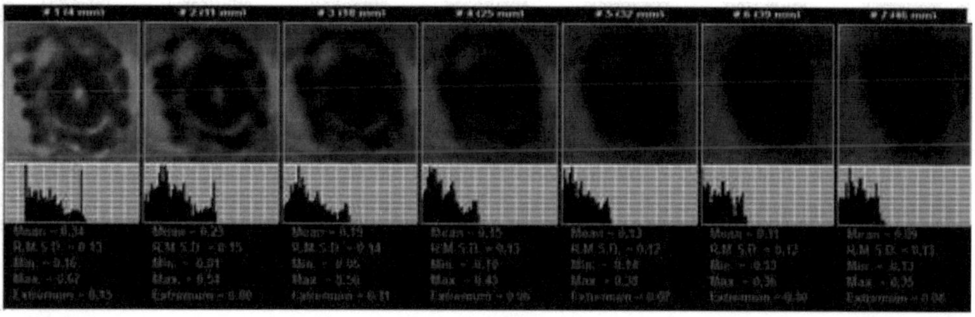

Figure 9. EIM. Seven scan planes. The mammary gland contour is distinct and without deformation.

- The areola is in the centre of the image, non-displaced, non-deformed, non-fragmented and coloured in black tones of greyscale (Figure 10).

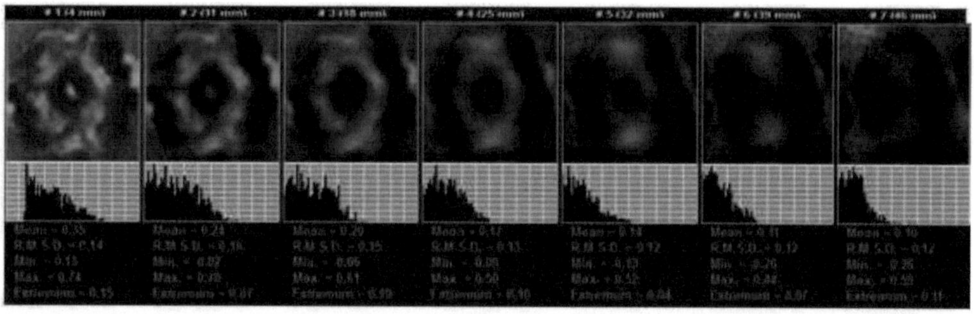

Figure 10. EIM. Seven scan planes. Central location of the areola. The areola is black.

- The mammary gland structure is represented by the parenchyma and the septa without focal changes (Figure 11).

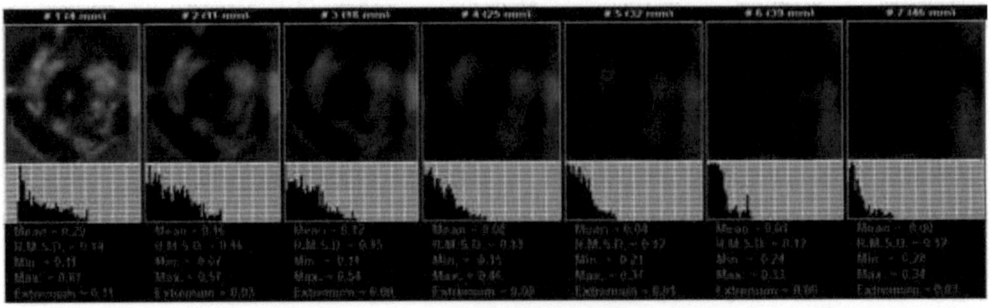

Figure 11. EIM. Seven scan planes. The parenchyma is without focal changes.

- The relative electrical conductivity of the left and right breasts is within normal range – the divergence of the electrical conductivity histograms is less than 20% (Figure 12).

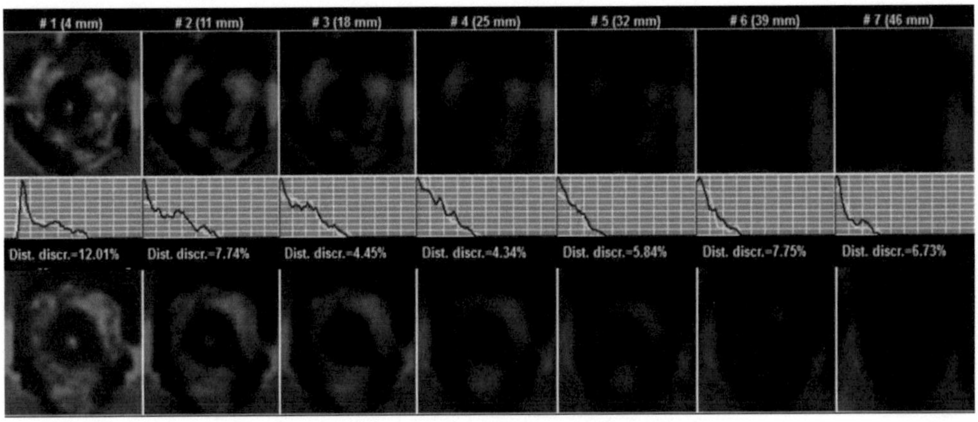

Figure 12. EIM. Seven scan planes. The top row shows images of the left breast, the bottom shows images of the right breast. The middle row presents a comparison of conductivity distribution histograms.

4.2. Normal mammographic scheme for amorphous-type breast structures

The predominance of an amorphous substance in the breast parenchyma structure can be observed among peri-menopausal and menopausal women. A considerable amount of fibrous friable connecting tissue in the mammary gland with a predominance of the basic substance helps the electric charge to pass. This conditions the characteristic features of the electrical impedance image: the predominance of lighter tones of greyscale; an absence of anatomic landmarks; high values of electrical conductivity. A normal electrical impedance mammographic scheme is expected to have all the characteristic features.

- The mammary gland contour is even and regular, without extrusions, retractions or unilateral thickening (Figure 13).

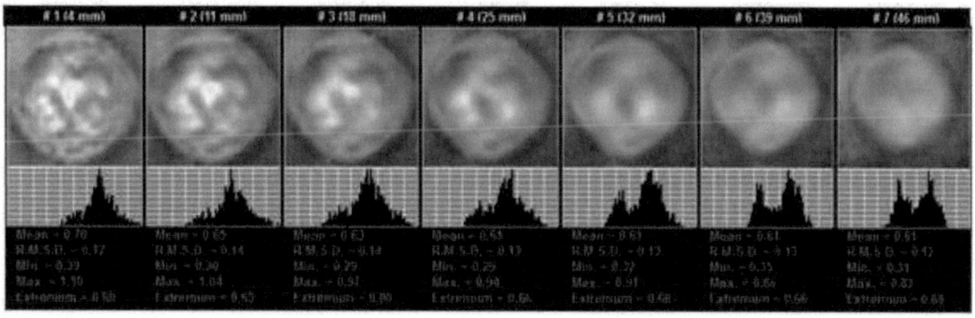

Figure 13. EIM. Seven scan planes. The mammary gland contour is distinct and without deformation.

- The areola is in the centre of the image, non-displaced, non-deformed, non-fragmented and coloured in white tones of greyscale (Figure 14).

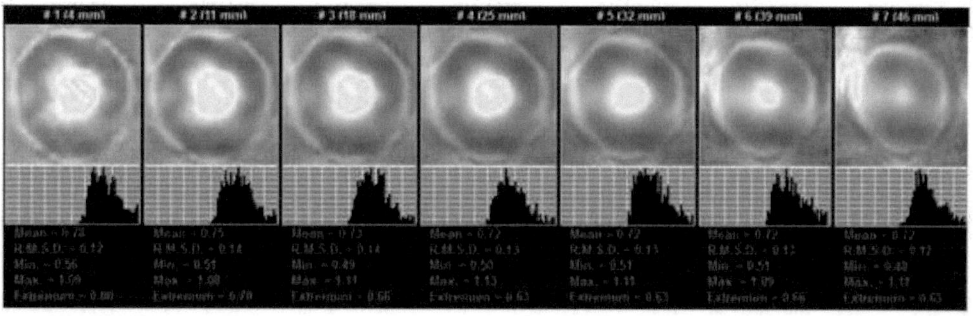

Figure 14. EIM. Seven scan planes. Central location of the areola. The areola is white.

- The mammary gland parenchyma is visualized as an unstructured mass, without septa and without focal changes (Figure 15).

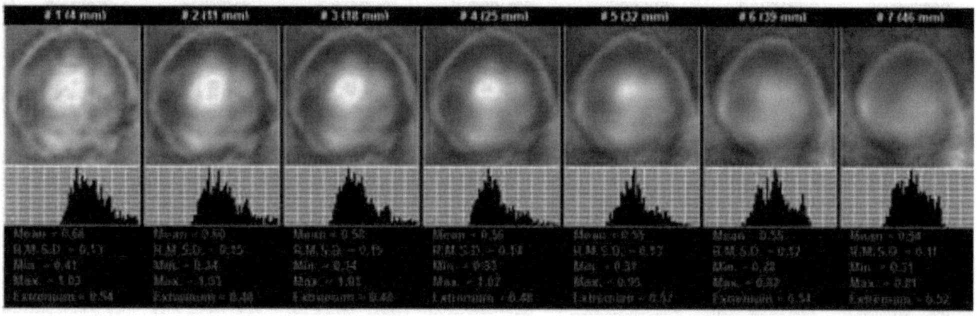

Figure 15. EIM. Seven scan planes. The parenchyma is without focal changes.

- The relative electrical conductivity of the left and right breasts is within normal range – the divergence of electrical conductivity histograms is less than 20% (Figure 16).

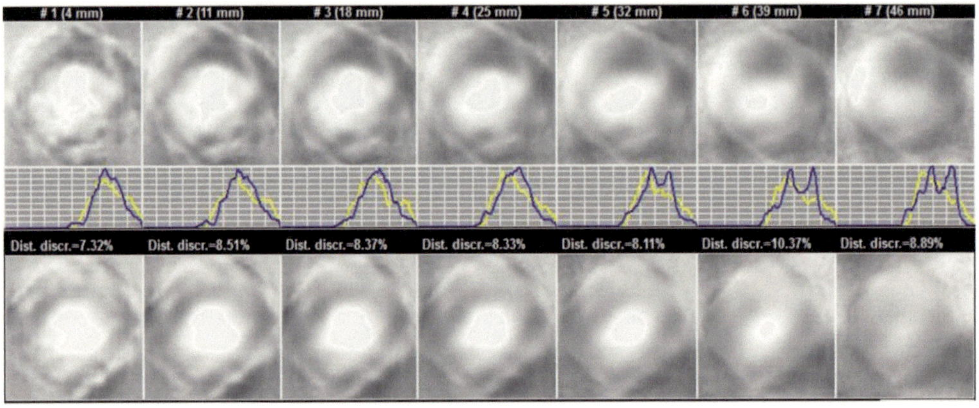

Figure 16. EIM. Seven scan planes. The top row shows images of the left breast, the bottom – of the right. The middle row demonstrates the comparison of conductivity distribution histograms.

4.3. Normal mammographic scheme for mixed-type breast structures

A mixed-type breast structure combines the elements of the ductal and amorphous types. Different combinations of these structures define the differing electrical conductivity of tissues and affect the electrical impedance image. The breast parenchyma becomes 'poorer' and homogeneous.

- The mammary gland contour is even and regular, without extrusions, retractions or unilateral thickening (Figure 17).

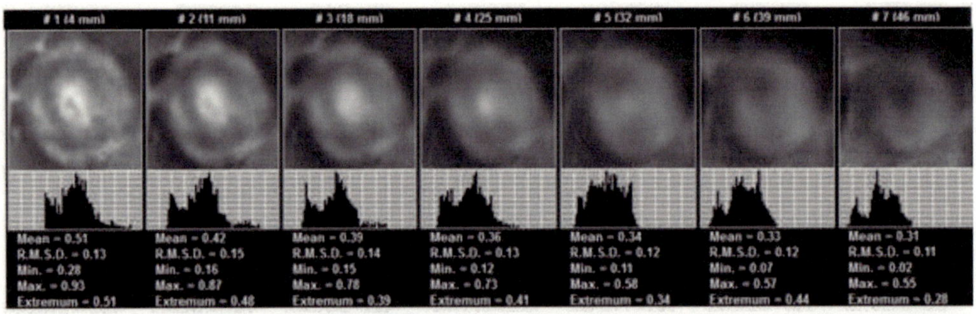

Figure 17. EIM. Seven scan planes. The mammary gland contour is distinct and without deformation

- The areola is in the centre of the figure, non-displaced, non-deformed, non-fragmented and the colour is variable (Figure 18).

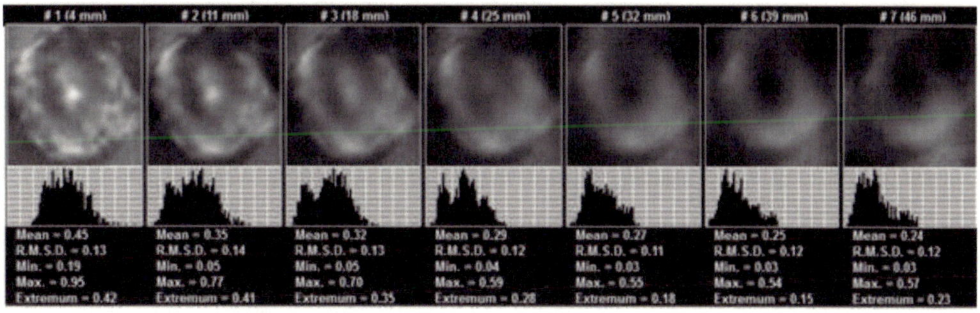

Figure 18. EIM. Seven scan planes. Central location of the areola.

- The mammary gland parenchyma is variable and without focal changes (Figure 19).

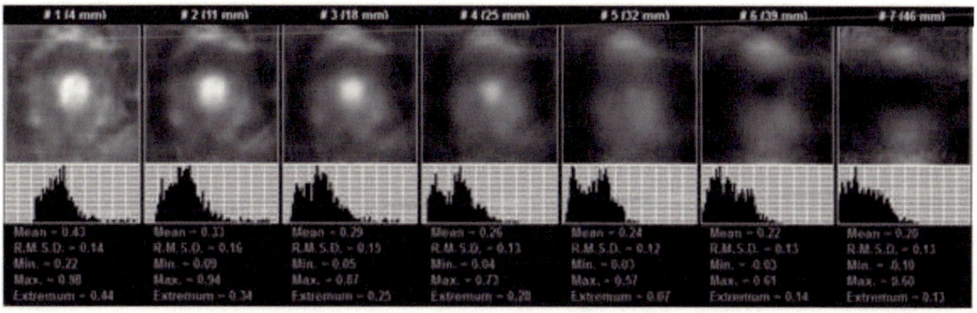

Figure 19. EIM. Seven scan planes. The parenchyma is without focal changes.

- The relative electrical conductivity of the left and right breasts is within normal range – the divergence of electrical conductivity histograms is less than 20% (Figure 20).

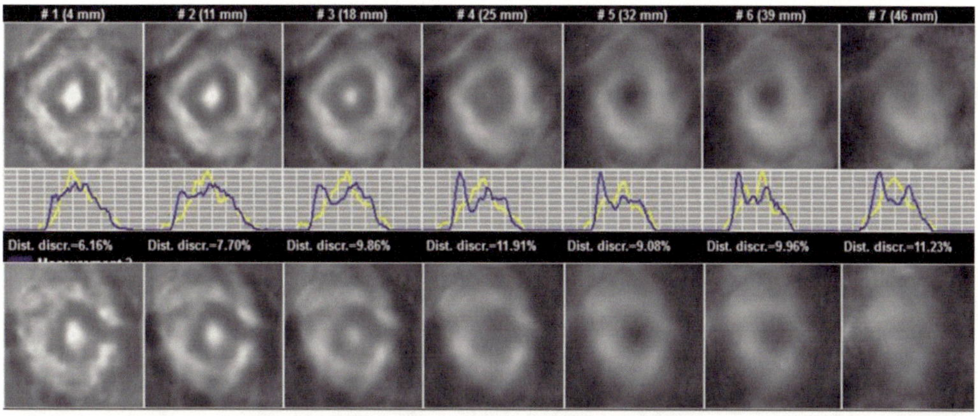

Figure 20. EIM. The top row shows images of the left breast, the bottom shows images of the right. The middle row demonstrates the comparison of the conductivity distribution histograms.

5. Electrical impedance mammographic scheme distortion in the presence of cancer

Here, we present the prospective assessment results of 310 cases of verified breast cancer. Electrical impedance mammograms were received from oncological centres in Russia, Belarus, South Africa and Malaysia. As a result, the mammographic scheme distortion was revealed in 74% of cases, whereas the change in the general electrical conductivity was detected in 67% of cases. Notably, this does not depend on the tumour size.

The assessment criteria of the mammographic scheme distortion included:

1. Alteration of the mammary gland contour

2. Alteration of the breast anatomy

3. Local electrical impedance alterations

4. Change of relative electrical conductivity

5.1. Mammary gland contour change

The visual assessment of the mammary gland image should start with the analysis of the breast contour. Usually, the contour of the mammary gland is even and regular, non-deformed and without an isoimpedance structure. In the presence of breast cancer, there is a chance of contour deformation and its hyperimpedance.

5.1.1. Contour deformation

Mammary gland contour deformation is an important diagnosis criterion in the presence of certain breast diseases. More often than not, deformation is caused by volumetric processes in the mammary gland, such as cancer. Cancer infiltration of tissues causes local contour deformations in the form of extrusion or retraction. In the top row, one can see images of a malignant breast with local contour deformation in the form of extrusion. The bottom row shows a tomogram of the normal breast (Figure 21).

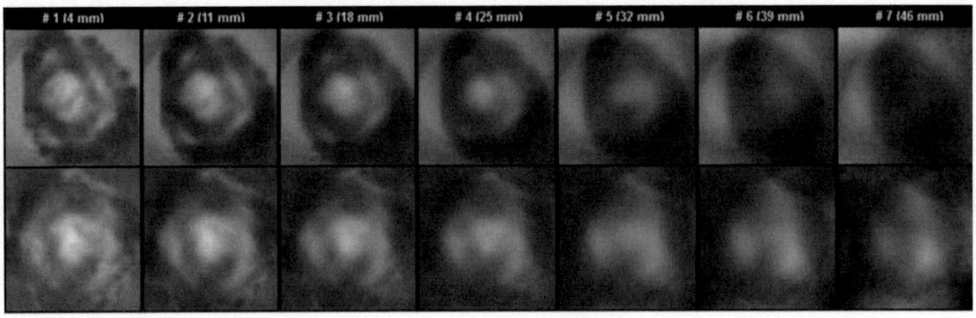

Figure 21. EIM. Seven scan planes. The top row shows images of a malignant breast.

http://dx.doi.org/10.5772/60014

A hyperimpedance contour with a protruding deformity is visible at 11 o'clock. The bottom row shows images of the normal breast.

5.1.2. *Thickening and hyperimpedance of the contour*

By contour hyperimpedance, one should understand a significant increase of electrical impedance on the periphery of the mammary gland. This phenomenon – unilateral as a rule – should be considered as a reaction of the breast tissues solely in response to a malignant process (Figure 22).

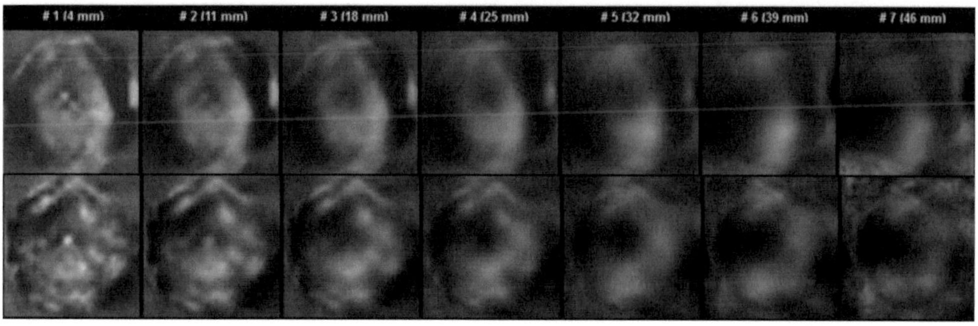

Figure 22. EIM. Seven scan planes. The top row shows images of a malignant breast. The bottom row shows images of the normal breast. A unilateral thickened hyperimpedance contour can clearly be seen.

In the electrical impedance image, a hyperimpedance contour is thickened and intensively black in colour. The top rows of the figures present tomograms with hyperimpedance contours of malignant breasts. In the bottom rows, tomograms of normal breasts are given. The contour hyperimpedance is revealed through the change in its colour and its significant thickening compared to the normal breast (Figure 23).

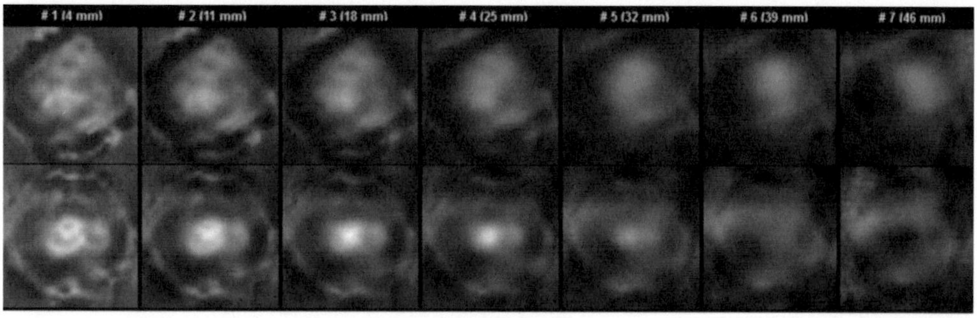

Figure 23. EIM. Seven scan planes. The top row shows images of a malignant breast. The bottom row shows images of the normal breast. A unilateral thickened hyperimpedance contour can be clearly seen.

5.2. Breast anatomy changes

Normally, an image of the mammary gland has an anatomy corresponding to the age-norm, with no shift of the inner structures.

In the presence of breast diseases, the breast anatomy undergoes changes. In Figures 24 and 25, we can clearly see the alteration of the mammary gland anatomy in the presence of cancer (top row) as compared to the images of the normal breast (bottom row).

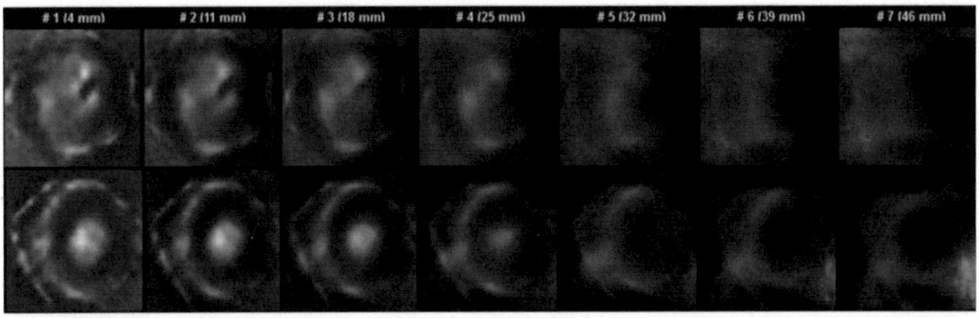

Figure 24. EIM. Seven scan planes. The top row shows images of a malignant breast, the bottom row shows images of the normal breast. A substantial change in the anatomy of the malignant breast accompanied by numerous hyperimpedance enclosures can clearly be seen.

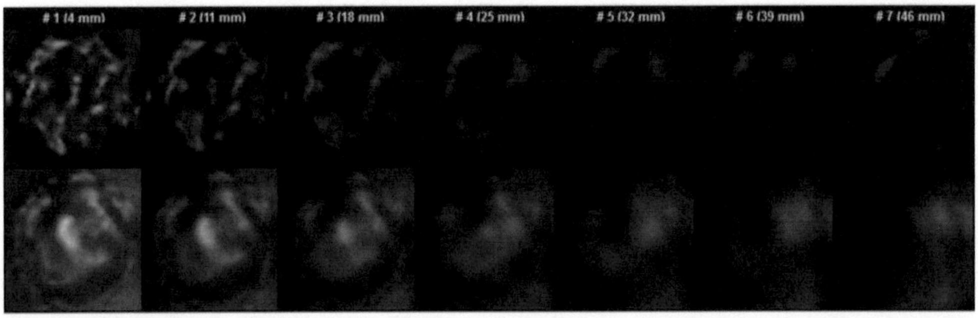

Figure 25. EIM. Seven scan planes. The top row shows images of a malignant breast, the bottom row shows images of the normal breast. No anatomic landmarks are visible in the malignant breast.

5.3. Local electrical conductivity changes

Some of the most important elements of image assessment are local electroconductivity changes outside the lacteous sinus area, and are uncommon in relation to the norm. In the presence of breast diseases, both areas with high impedance (i.e., hyperimpedance area) and areas with low impedance (i.e., hypoimpedance area) can be visualized.

5.3.1. *Local hyperimpedance*

This figure presents an image of a malignant breast. A focal change of electric conductivity in the form of a non-homogeneous hyperimpedance area with sharp contours and local contour-thickening is visible at eight o'clock. Such changes are typical of an infiltrative process. The bottom row shows images of the normal breast (Figure 26).

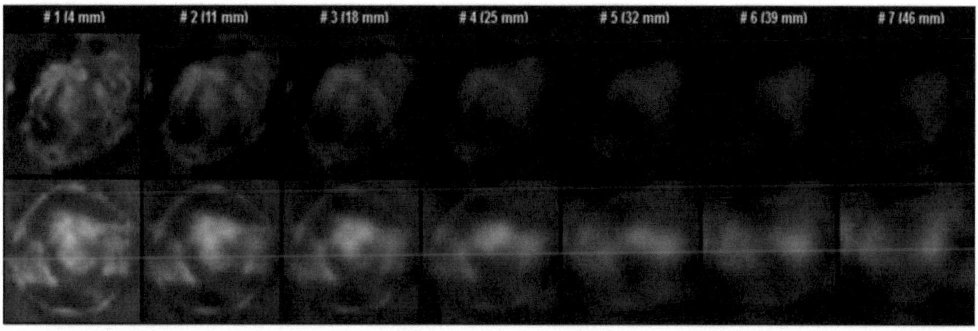

Figure 26. EIM. Seven scan planes. The top row shows images of a malignant breast. A focal change of electric conductivity in the form of a non-homogeneous hyperimpedance area is visible at eight o'clock. The bottom row shows images of the normal breast.

5.3.2. *Local hypoimpedance*

Focal changes of electric conductivity in the form of a hypoimpedance area with indistinct contours are visible at 11 o'clock. This is also typical of cancer (Figure 27).

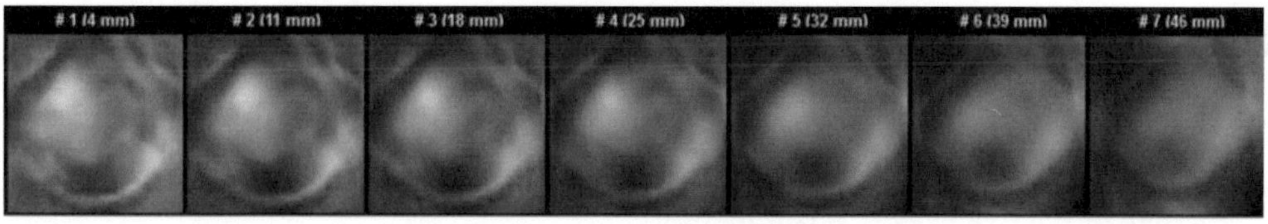

Figure 27. EIM. Seven scan planes. Focal changes of electric conductivity in the form of a hypoimpedance area with indistinct contours are visible at 11 o'clock.

In addition, in the presence of breast cancer, a hyperimpedance contour can be visualized around the infiltration zone. The top row shows images of the malignant breast. A focal change of electric conductivity visualizing itself as an irregularly-shaped area with a hyperimpedance contour and a hypoimpedance structure can be found at two o'clock. The bottom row shows images of the normal breast (Figure 28).

5.3.3. *Total hyperimpedance*

There are cases of electrical conductivity disturbance that reveal themselves as total impedance increases. This can be observed during the infiltrative oedematous form of breast cancer. In

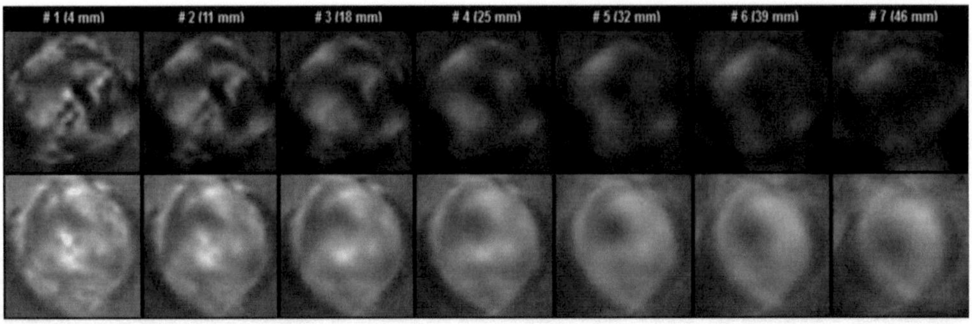

Figure 28. EIM. Seven scan planes. The top row shows images of a malignant breast. A focal change of electric conductivity visualizing itself as an irregularly-shaped area with a hyperimpedance contour and a hypoimpedance structure can be found at two o'clock. The bottom row shows images of the normal breast.

the figures, the top row presents a breast with total high impedance, which is common for cancer. In the bottom row, there is a tomogram of a normal breast (Figure 29).

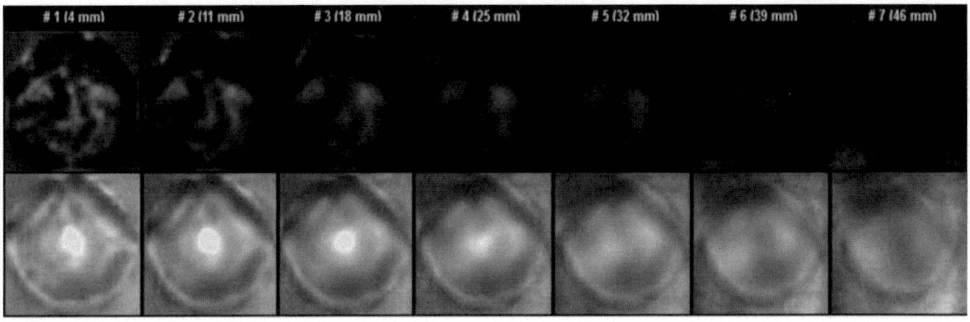

Figure 29. EIM. Seven scan planes. The top row shows images of a malignant breast. The bottom row shows images of a normal breast. The image of the malignant breast is domineered by hyperimpedance tones due to the decrease in electric conductivity.

5.4. Change of relative electrical conductivity

Unlike other methods of visualization, the electrical impedance method makes the quantitative analysis of the image possible. The quantitative analysis of the electrical impedance image implies the assessment of the following parameters: mean electrical conductivity index; histogram of conductivity distribution; comparison with the reference data. To attribute patients to a certain class (healthy or diseased), we have applied the following: the criterion of difference in the form of distributions; the λ criterion; the Kholmogorov-Smirnov criterion (or the DX statistics); an intermediate index in Kholmogorov-Smirnov's computations. This criterion, relating to nonparametric criteria, allows the assessment of the statistical significance of divergences in the distribution of any mark of the norm or pathology, including the electrical conductivity distribution on electrical impedance tomograms. The Dx statistics permit the assessment of the surface of one of the distributions which is not common with the second distribution. The Dx value reflects the share of observations or data which distinguish the

http://dx.doi.org/10.5772/60014

experience (patient) from the control (norm) group. This value is important, both for the substantiation of the diagnosis and the assessment of the information value of the index. A high informative value of differences revealed allows the attribution of the patient to one class or another (e.g., norm or cancer). In order to determine the informative capacity of distribution divergence, we used the information measure of S. Kullback, which demonstrated the informativity of the applied Dx statistics and the input of this index in disease diagnosis, for example, cancer. The assessment of the distribution divergence yielded results which are in direct dependency on the value according to S. Kullback [9] (Table 2).

Distribution divergence	Informative value	Reliability
Up to 20%	very low	no
20-30%	relatively low	yes
30-50%	good	yes
50-65%	high	yes
70-85%	extremely high	yes

Table 2. Informative content and accuracy for different values (%) of conductivity distribution diversion.

In the presence of diseases, mammary gland histogram offset takes place (Figure 30).

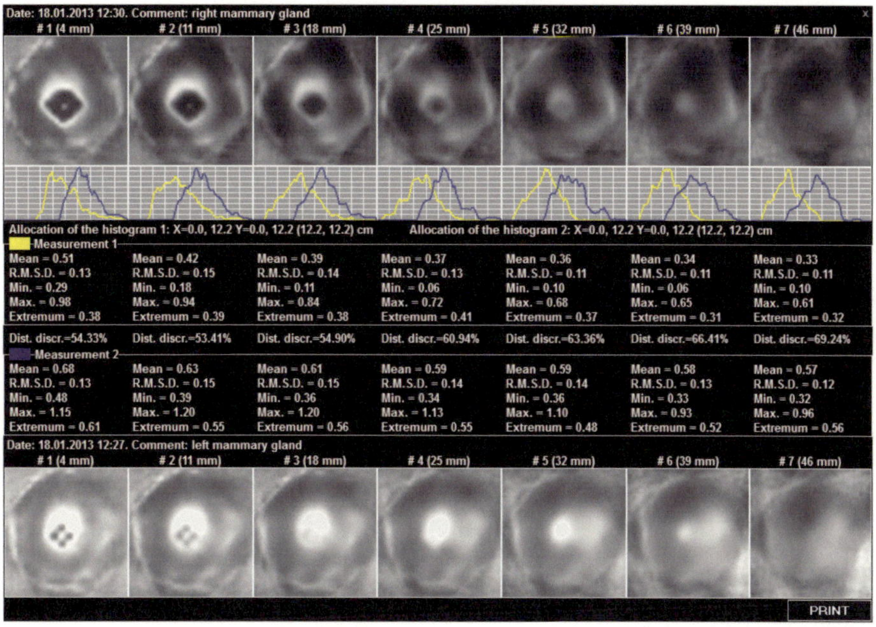

Figure 30. Upper row – EIM. Seven scan planes. Breast cancer. Bottom row - EIM. Seven scan planes. Healthy gland. The second row shows the divergence between the histograms of the electrical conductivity distribution of the affected and healthy glands.Table 3, below, contains the data on the relative conductivity of malignant breasts as compared to breasts undergoing benign changes, normal breasts and breasts with different anatomies.

	Number of patients	Relative conductivity (diseased - healthy mammary gland)					
		< 20%	20-30%	30-40%	40-50%	50-60%	>60%
Cancer	310	101 (33%)	67 (22%)	44 (14%)	37 (12%)	26 (8%)	35 (11%)
Healthy	161	157 (98%)	4 (2%)	0	0	0	0
Healthy Acinal/ductal-type mammary gland structure.	20	18 (90%)	1 (5%)	1 (5%)	0	0	0
Healthy Amorphous-type mammary gland structure.	32	28 (88%)	2 (6%)	2 (6%)	0	0	0
Benign	68	59 (87%)	7 (10%)	2 (3%)	0	0	0

Table 3. Relative breast conductivity for the norm and pathology.

As the oncological process develops, the overall and local conductivity changes. At the same time, the distortion of the normal mammographic scheme can already be observed at the initial stages of the disease. It is for this reason that the given criterion is included in the EIM scale of breast cancer diagnosis (Table 4).

Diagnostic criteria	Electrical impedance mammography points
Shape	
• round, oval	1
• lobular, irregular	2
Contour	
• no	0
• sharp	1
• hyperimpedance, indistinct	2
Surrounding tissues	
• preserved	0
• structure alteration/displacement	1
• thickening/extrusion/retraction	2
Internal electrical structure	
• hyperimpedance ($IC_{roi}<IC_{av}+2std$)	0
• isoimpedance $IC_{roi}=IC_{av}\pm2std$)	1
• hypoimpedance ($IC_{roi}>IC_{av}+2std$)	2
• animpedance ($IC_{roi}>IC_{av}+3std$)	3

Diagnostic criteria	Electrical impedance mammography points
Comparative electrical conductivity	
• divergence between the histograms < 20%	0
• divergence between the histograms 20-30 %	1
• divergence between the histograms 30-40%	2
• divergence between the histograms > 40%	3

Table 4. Diagnostic criteria for differentiating volumetric lesions in electrical impedance mammography.

6. Conclusion

The alteration of the normal mammographic scheme along with the abnormal changes of local conductivity is one of the early diagnostic criteria for breast cancer.

Electrical impedance mammography represents a method allowing the formation of observation and risk groups for the development of breast cancer through the use of data on relative electrical conductivity and the age-related electrical conductivity scale.

Complications of the oncological process with oedema are a serious obstacle for X-ray and US diagnostics. Unlike the aforementioned methods of diagnosis, electrical impedance tomography makes it possible to visualize pathophysiological changes in such states as cancer, mastitis and lymphostasis, etc.

Author details

Alexander Karpov[1*], Andrey Kolobanov[2] and Marina Korotkova[1]

*Address all correspondence to: karpovay@medyar.ru

1 Clinical Hospital #9, Yaroslavl, Russia

2 Railroad Clinical Hospital, Yaroslavl, Russia

References

[1] Boyd NF, Byng JW, Jong RA, Fishell EK, Little LE, Miller AB, Lockwood GA, Tritcher DL, Yaffe MJ. Quantitative classification of mammographic densities and breast cancer risk: results from Canadian National Breast Screening Study. *J. Natl. Cancer Inst.* 1995; 87; 670-675.

[2] Wolfe JN, Saftias AF, Salane M. Mammographic parenchymal patterns and quantitative evaluation of mammographic densities: a case-control study. *AJR Am J Roentgenol.* 1987, 148, 1087-1092.

[3] American College of Radiology. BI-RADS Breast Imaging Reporting and Data System. Virginia: Reston; 2003.

[4] Electrical Impedance Tomography. IOP, 2005.

[5] Cherepenin V, Karpov A, Korjenevsky A, Kornienko V, Mazaletskaya A, Mazurov D. A 3D electrical impedance tomography (EIT) system for breast cancer detection. *Physiological Measurement.* 2001, 22, 9-18.

[6] Karpov A, Korjenevsky A, Mazurov D, Mazaletskaya A. 3D Electrical Impedance Scanning of Breast Cancer. *World Congress on Medical Physics and Biomedical Engineering, Chicago,* 2000, 62.

[7] Dunaeva O, Gerasimov D, Karpov A, Machin M, Tchayev A, Tsofin Yu, Tsyplyonkov V. Using Backprojection Algorithm for 3D Image Reconstruction in EIT. *World Congress on Medical Physics and Biomedical Engineering,* Munich, Germany, 2009.

[8] Korotkova M, Karpov A. Procedure for assessment of the mammary gland electrical impedance images. *XIII international conference on electrical bio-impedance.* Graz, Austria, 2007.

[9] Gubler E. Quantitative methods for analysis and identification of pathology. Leningrad, 1978.

Chapter 2

Ultrasound Axillary Imaging

Nastasia Serban

Additional information is available at the end of the chapter

http://dx.doi.org/10.5772/59730

1. Introduction

The most significant prognostic factors in breast cancer are the tumoral diameter, tumor grading and the status of the axillary lymph nodes. The presence of nodal metastases decreases 5-year survival by approximately 40% compared to node-negative patients, in reference [1]. Lymph node status is of particular value in choosing further therapy. Lymph node metastatic disease is an indication for skipping sentinel node biopsy (SLNB) (and proceeding to complete axillary dissection) and/or for adjuvant systemic chemotherapy, which may be of benefit if administered as preoperative treatment.

2. The anatomy of the axillary lymph node

The anatomy of the axillary lymph node includes the cortex and the medulla. The high-frecquency probes allow the differentiation of the central echogenic hilum and the peripheral hypoechoic cortex. The cortex, which includes the marginal sinus and the lymphoid follicles is hypoechoic and thin, and has a fusiform shape with smooth edge. The hilum is the hyperechoic, its echogenity being attributable to multiple reflective interfaces of blood vessels, fat, and the central sinus, in reference [2,3].

Carcinoma from the breast enters the lymph node via the afferent lymphatics, penetrates the capsule, and enters the subcapsular sinus, in reference [4]. Metastatic cells firstly stop in the periphery (cortex) of the nodes, causing cortical enlargement. Then generalized cortical enlargement and destruction of the nodal architecture occurs, with compression and, eventually, loss of the hilum, in reference [2].

3. Assessment of axillary lymph nodes status

Grossly involvement of axillary lymph nodes can be detected by clinical examination, ultrasound or axilla MRI. However, introduction of screening mammography led to earlier diagnosis of breast cancer, in which axillary involvement is frequently absent. The challenge of imaging technique is to differentiate the normal lymph nodes from the nodes with minimal metastatic disease, which do not change the size and shape of the lymph node, in patients with small primary breast tumors.

The "golden standard" for axillary lymph node status is pathological examination of lymph nodes. There are three possibilities to obtain information regarding the axillary lymph nodes status: complete axillary lymph node dissection, biopsy of the sentinel lymph node (SLN) and pretreatment imaging of the axillary lymph nodes, associated or not with fine-needle aspiration cytology or core biopsy of the suspicious nodes.

Complete lymph node dissection represents the classic approach that allows pathological examination of all the lymph nodes in the axilla. However, complete axillary lymph node dissection is accompanied by complications like seroma formation, numbness, limitation of shoulder movement, and lymphedema, in reference [5].

SLN biopsy (SLNB) represents the biopsy of that lymph node, which first collects the lymph from the breast. It is a surgical procedure, requiring preoperative administration of a dye and/ or radionuclide tracer.

Pretreatment imaging of the axillary lymph nodes must closely match the pathological findings in order to have any value for clinical decision making. Many studies suggest that patients with axillary involvement may benefit from preoperative systemic treatment. Imaging techniques for axilla include ultrasound, MRI enhanced or nonenhanced, FDG-PET scan, 99mTc-sestamibi scintigraphy.

4. Ultrasound evaluation of axilla

The most available imaging technique for axilla is ultrasound. Ultrasound has two roles in visualizing the axilla: a) to characterize the abnormal lymph nodes, either identified by US or by clinical examination or other imaging technique and b) to help axillar SLN identification. In both circumstances, ultrasound helps the biopsy of the nodes.

Afferent lymphatic channels enter a node through the periphery of the cortex, so the malignant cells travelling the lymphatic vessel will first stop in the cortical region of the lymph node. Most of the US signs of lymph nodes metastasis will refer to the abnormalities of the cortex. Subtle abnormalities of the cortex can indicate early metastatic involvement.

For the assessment of a lymph node by US, quantitative or qualitative methods have been used.

4.1. The qualitative features of a metastatic lymph node on US

The qualitative features of a metastatic lymph node on US include shape (round morphology), asymmetric cortical thickening (Figure 1), loss of central hilum, loss or compression of the hyperechoic medullary region (Figure 2), relationship with neighbouring lymph nodes, left-to-right asimetry and increased peripheral blood flow. Even more, lymph nodes can exhibit ultrasound malignancy signs characteristic to the primary breast tumor, such as angular margins, „taller than wide" (Figure 3) or they appears intensely vascularisated on Doppler ultrasound. Reactive changes associated with inflamation produce an increase of blood flux in the preexisting blood vessels, but do not generate new vessel formation or vessels that can penetrate the capsule. Metastatic disease stimulates new vessels formation, so Doppler examination can reveal an intense Doppler signal inside the lymph node or blood vessel penetrating the capsule.

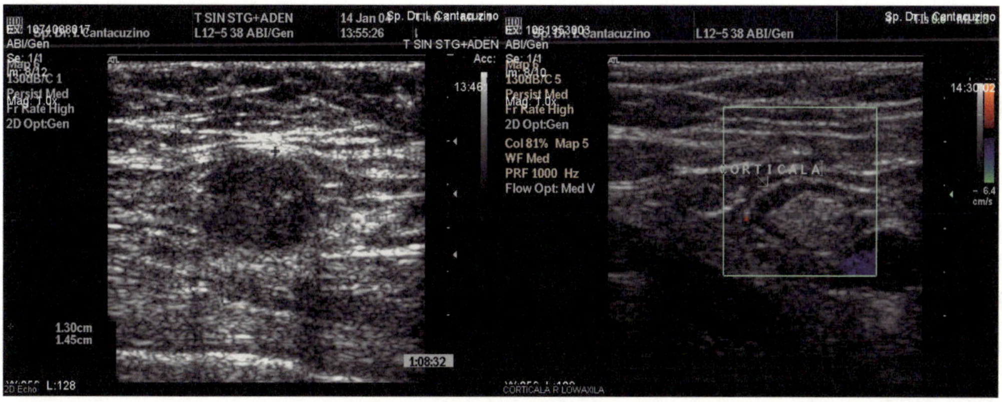

Figure 1. Left: Metastatic lymph node, with a round shape. Invasive ductal carcinoma (primary tumor of 1.8 cm, three SLNs identified, all of them metastatic, and complete axillary dissection). Right: asymmetrical cortical thickening in a metastatic axillary lymph node (with normal the cortex-hilum area ratio).

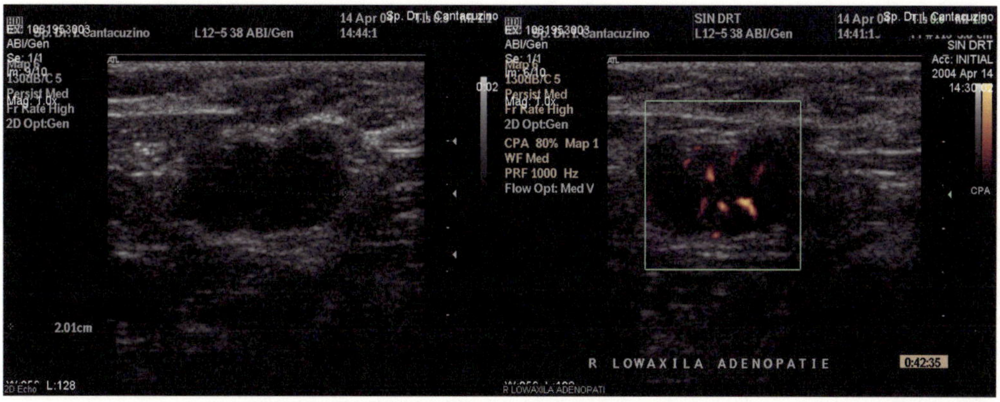

Figure 2. Metastatic lymph node. Left: loss of the hyperechoic medullary region. Right: on power Doppler examination, this node is displaying both central and peripheral blood flow.

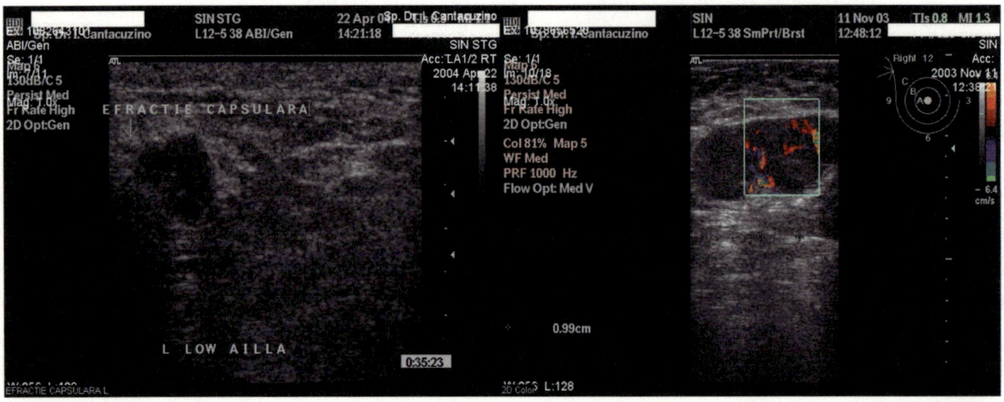

Figure 3. Left, metastatic lymphadenopathy, exhibiting „taller than wide" property and angular margins. Pathology showed capsular efraction. Right, gigantic metastatic lymphadenopathy with increased vascularisation and intact capsule.

4.2. The quantitative indicators of a metastatic lymph node on US

The quantitative indicators of a metastatic lymph node on US include the size (Figure 4, left), maximum thickness of the cortex, in reference [6] (Figure 4, right; Figure 5), the cortex-hilum (CH) area ratio, in reference [7] (Figure 5), the longitudinal-transverse (LT) axis ratio, in reference [7], the number of peripheral blood vessels.

Lymph nodes can be enlarged, either by metastatic disease or reactive changes, including fat degeneration. Reactive changes in lymph nodes increase all dimensions, keeping the eliptical shape and a normal cortical/medullar index. Metastatic disease will increase the lymph node small diameter, will replace the medullar hyperechogenic region with hypoechogenic tumoral tissue, so the maximum thickness of the cortex and cortex-hilum area ratio will increase, eventually completely destroying the hilum (absent hilum).

A small study of the author, in reference [8], evaluating 21 consecutive breast cancer patients, in which SLNB was performed, suggest that ultrasound size > 1 cm of lymph nodes correlates with invasion of SLN (Figure 4, left).

Cortical region evaluation is more important in lymph nodes assessment than size. The absolute cortical thickness is predictive for axillary metastatic disease (Figure 4, right), a cortical thickness more than 2.5 mm being associated in 70 percent of cases with lymph node metastasis (Cho N et al, 2009, in reference [6]).

Song SE et al, in reference [7], evaluated the diagnostic performance for their own positive criteria for lymph node metastasis, such as CH area ratio >2 (Figure 5), LT axis ratio <2 or peripheral type of vascularisation on power Doppler imaging. They found that the sensitivity of the CH area ratio was superior to that of the LT axis ratio (94.1% vs. 82.3%, p=0.031) and to that of the peripheral blood flow pattern (94.1% vs. 29.4%, p=0.009) (Figure 6). For specificity, all three parameters had the same high values (89.1-95.6%; NS).

http://dx.doi.org/10.5772/59730

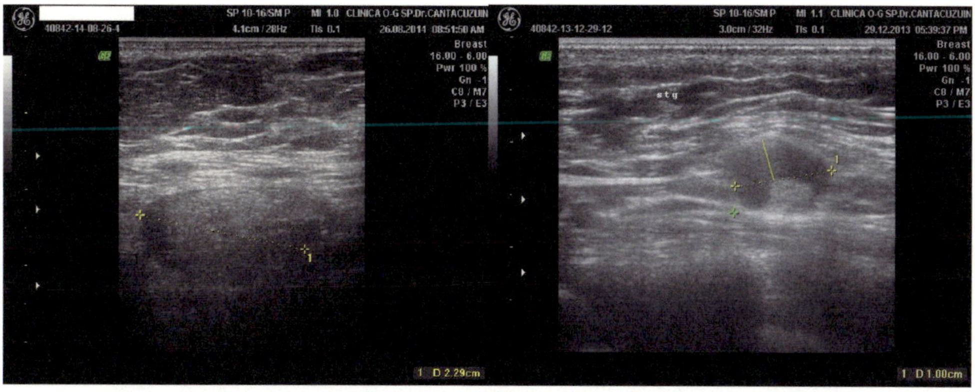

Figure 4. Left: metastatic lymph node, showing increased size (longest dimension of 2,29 cm), in a case of advanced invasive ductal carcinoma. Core biopsy of this node showed invasive duct carcinoma. Right: maximum thickness of the cortex of 4 mm in a metastatic lymph node (invasive ductal carcinoma).

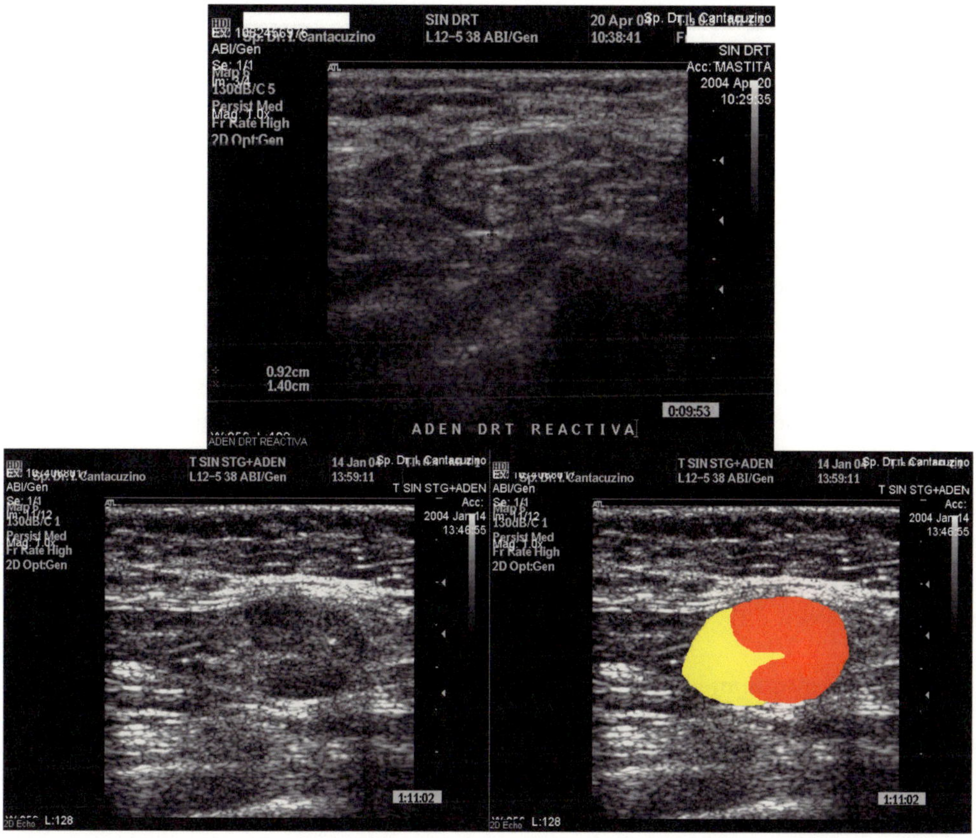

Figure 5. Above: reactive lymphadenopathy in patient with postpartum mastitis. There is moderate and simetrical increase of cortical thickness, but normal cortical/medullar index. Below: metastatic axillary lymph node with cortical/medullar index of 1.82 and an absolute increase of cortical thickness > 2.5 mm.

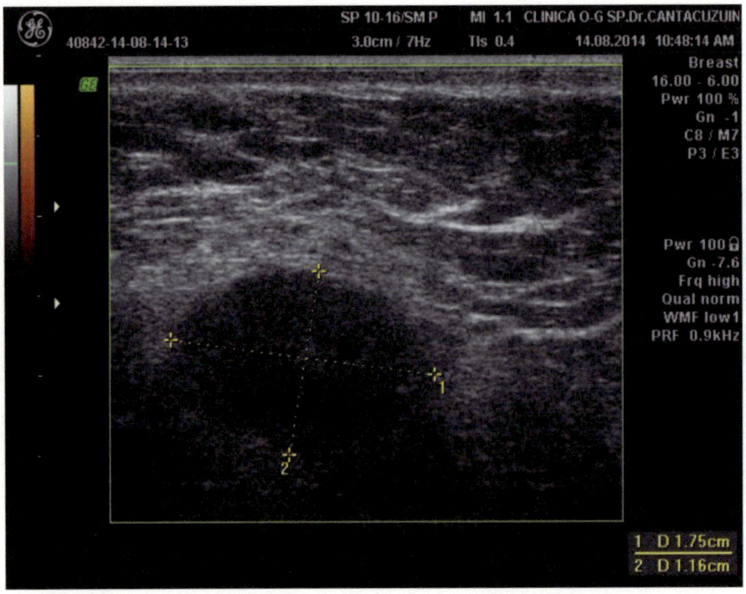

Figure 6. Metastatic axillary lymph node with LT axis ratio of 1.50; blood flow was absent on power Doppler.

4.3. Sonoelastography

Sonoelastography can be added to axillary lymph nodes ultrasound evaluation for further increase the precision of identification of metastatic lymph nodes. At present, there are not many studies trying to establish the place of sonoelastography in evaluation of axillary lymph nodes status. Choi (2011, 64 patients, in reference [9]), Taylor (2011, 50 patients, in reference [10]), Wojcinski (2012, 180 patients, in reference [11]) found that sonoelastography is capable of detecting elasticity differences between the cortex and medulla, and between metastatic and healthy LNs.

Wojcinski et al (2012) found that the highest sensibility (73.3%) is obtained when cortex >3mm in B-mode OR blue cortex in the elastogram, while, when these two features are found together (cortex >3mm in B-mode AND blue cortex in the elastogram (Figure 7)), the highest specificity is obtained (99.3%).

4.4. The role of ultrasound in sentinel lymph node identification and biopsy

Ultrasound has a role in sentinel lymph node identification. With introduction of indocyanine green for sentinel lymph node biopsy (SLNB), Tagaya et al (2010) were able to visualize the fluorescence of lymphatic vessels on the skin. The authors performed firstly intraoperative ultrasonography to identify a SLN as the first lymph node recognized during ultrasonography scanning from the edge of the breast gland in the direction of the axilla and they marked its position on the axillary skin. After indocyanine green dye injection, lymphatic ducts were visualized towards the axilla and the fluorescence stream disappeared aproximatively 1 cm

http://dx.doi.org/10.5772/59730

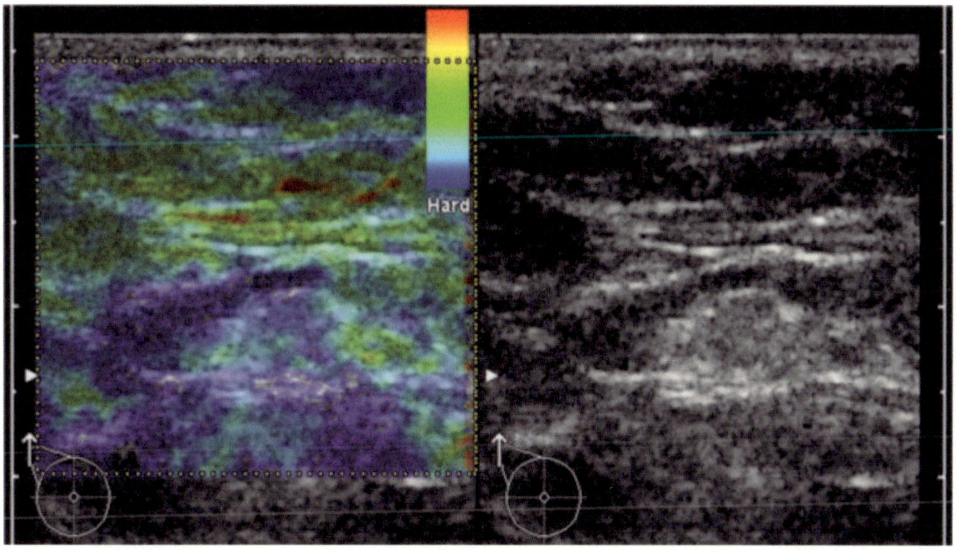

Figure 7. Wojcinski et al, 2012, in reference [11]. Open Access. Example for B-mode ultrasound and elastogram of a metastatic LN. In B-mode ultrasound, the cortex of the LN is slightly enlarged (maximum ~3.5mm). The predominant color of the medulla is turquoise (to green) and the cortex is mainly blue. Meeting both criteria of cortex >3mm in B-mode AND blue cortex in the elastogram, this case would be a true-positive.

before the line marked on the skin for ultrasound SLN location. In this study, the sites of skin incision for SLNB were also identical with the LN that had been demonstrated by ultrasonography in all patients.

Ultrasound signs of SLN involvement could be very subtle, with only a minimal focal cortical thickness increase.

By recognizing the first lymph node during scanning towards axilla (Figure 8), ultrasound may help SLN identification and decrease the operation time, an important fact because as the identification time increase, more SLNs are found.

However, in case of axillary metastases, identification of SLN may be impaired (Esen G, Gurses B, 2005, in [12]).

4.5. The role of ultrasound in imagistic staging of breast cancer

Ultrasound could have a role in imagistic staging of breast cancer. Knowledge of axillary lymph node involvement before surgery may allow for individualization of multimodal treatment. This may include preoperative chemotherapy, intraoperative breast radiotherapy or plastic surgery for immediate reconstruction.

The future protocols of breast cancer treatment will probably include ultrasound as a step in preoperative sentinel node mapping. Ultrasound may reveal abnormalities of axillary lymph nodes and guide biopsy of these nodes.

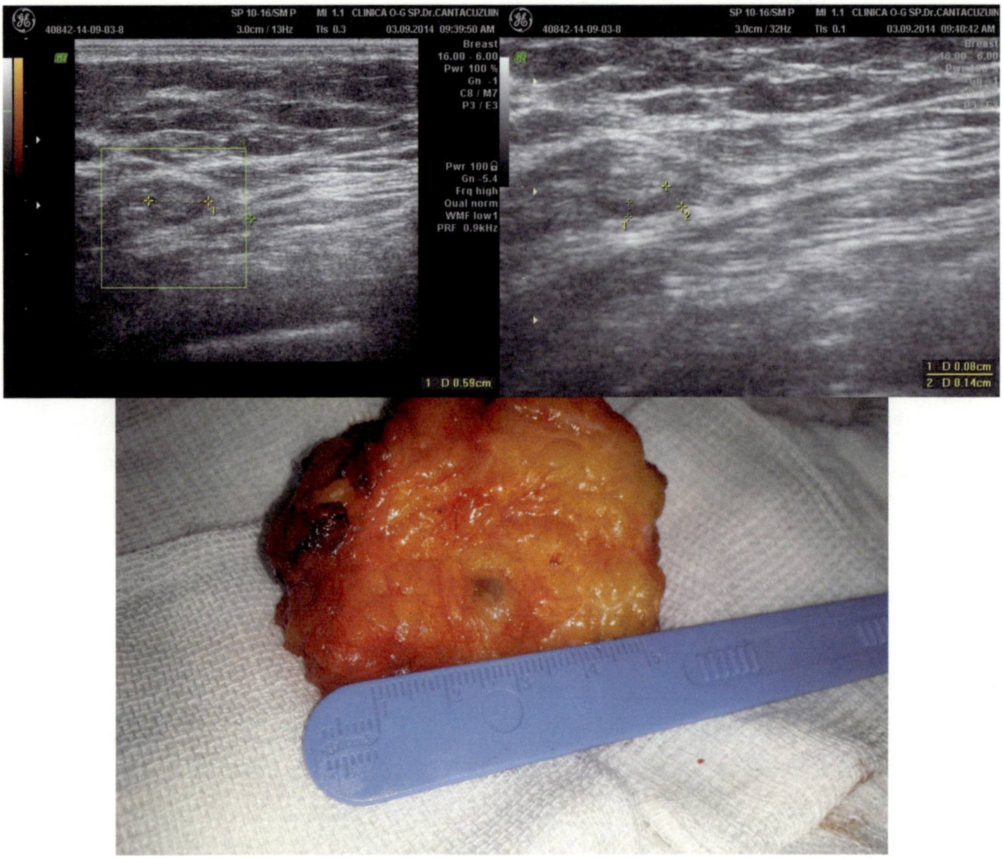

Figure 8. Above: preoperative assessment of axilla in a breast cancer patient with preoperative chemotherapy. The first lymph node during scanning towards axilla: sentinel lymph node with normal size (longest dimension 5.9 mm) and shape, but with smal focal cortical thickness. Below: intraoperative identification of SLN. After complete axillary dissection, the sentinel lymph and all the other nodes were negative.

Patients with either normal or abnormal ultrasound exams, but negative cytology, underwent sentinel node mapping. Patients with abnormal ultrasound and positive cytology proceeded to complete axillary dissection, in reference [13].

There are studies trying to assess the tumoral burden in patient with positive nodes. The study of Moore A et al, in [13], indicates that abnormalities limited to the lymph node cortex (Figure 9) were indicative of N1 disease.

Ultrasound features of axilla, suggesting metastasis in lymph nodes, combined with results of cytology or biopsy, could modify the surgical approach to the axilla, eliminating the need for sentinel node mapping in a significant proportion of patients, in reference [13].

Loss or compression of the hyperechoic medullary region, absence of fatty hilum, abnormal lymph node shape and increased peripheral blood flow are predictive of N2–3 disease, in reference [13] (Figure 10).

http://dx.doi.org/10.5772/59730

Preoperative ultrasound associated with ultrasound-guided biopsy can be used for preoperative axillary staging in patients who will be referred to preoperative systemic therapy. Study of Joh et al, in reference [14], showed that planning and initiation of preoperative systemic therapy can reliably be done using ultrasound axillary evaluation and biopsy.

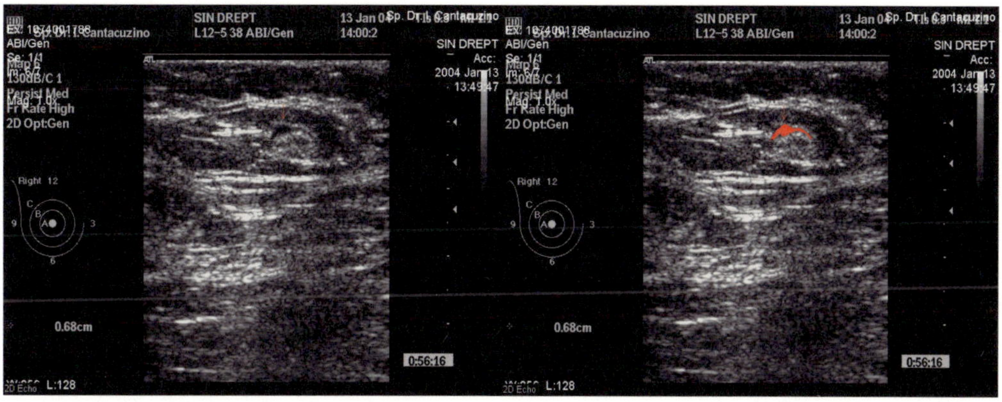

Figure 9. Postoperative assessment of ultrasound. The first lymph node during scanning towards axilla: metastatic sentinel lymph node with normal size and shape, but with smal focal cortical thickness. After complete axillary dissection, the sentinel lymph node was the only metastatic lymph node.

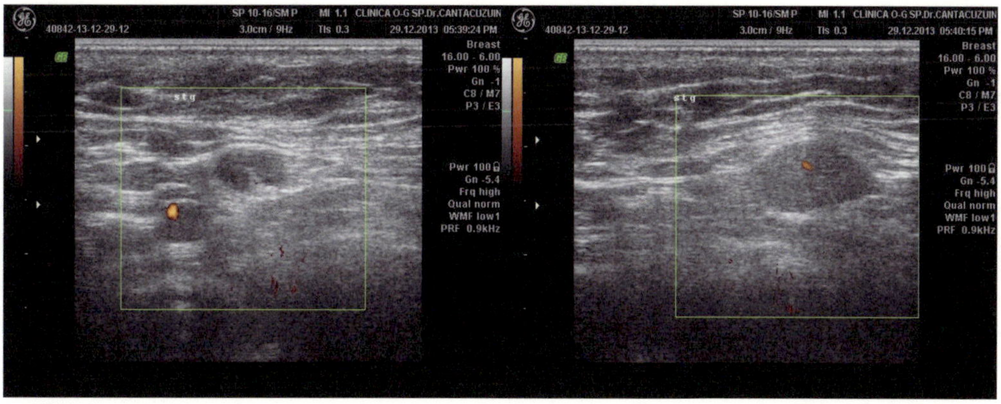

Figure 10. Left and right: same case – advanced ductal carcinoma (T3 N2 M0). Three lymph nodes displaying the features of metastatic disease. Axillary metastases were confirmed by core biopsy, and the patient was referred to preoperative chemotherapy.

4.6. Percutaneous biopsy procedures

Unfortunetly, no imaging technique has enough reliability to attribute patients directly to complete axillary dissection, without first performing SLNB. The study of Valente SA, Sener

SF et al, in [15], evaluated retrospectively 244 consecutive patients diagnosed with invasive breast carcinoma, by physical examination of the axilla, digital mammography, axillary ultrasonography, and contrast enhanced breast magnetic resonance imaging. The authors found that from the patients who had all four modalities negative, 14% were ultimately found to have histologically positive nodes at the time of surgery.

The role of ultrasound in staging breast cancer differs with stage of disease, helping treatment decisions for surgery, chemotherapy, and radiation therapy.

4.6.1. Percutaneous biopsy procedures in operable breast cancer

In operable breast cancer, ultrasound helps identification of sentinel lymph node and of suspicious nodes, that warrant biopsy. Ultrasound alone has modest accuracy in detecting axillary metastasis, not being reliable, on its own, to make a decision in surgical treatment of the axilla. Ultrasound does not provide enough information to refer patients to complete axillary dissection.

The reported a median ultrasound sensitivity, in a meta-analysis of 21 studies, including 4313 patients, made by Houssami et al, was 61.4% [51.2%-79.4%], and the median ultrasound specificity was 82.0% (76.9%-89.0%), in reference [16]. Adding a axillary biopsy procedure to ultrasound, to assess patients with abnormal or suspicious axillary nodes, leads to a good sensitivity and excellent specificity (nearly 100%). The same meta-analysis, made by Houssami et al, in [16], evaluated 1733 patients, in whom needle biopsy was added and guided by ultrasound, because of abnormal findings. In these patients, the ultrasound-guided biopsy had median sensitivity of 79.4% (68.3%-8.9%) and a median specificity of 100% (100%-100%).

The study of Holwit DM, Margenthaler JA, in [17], retrospectively performed on 256 patients with clinically node-negative breast cancer, who underwent axillary ultrasound (AUS) evaluation and ultrasound-guided FNAB/needle core biopsy only in suspicious-appearing lymph nodes, found that the sensitivity and specificity of axillary ultrasound alone were 79% and 81%, respectively. The overall combined sensitivity and specificity for AUS-guided FNAB/needle core biopsy were 71% and 99%, respectively, with a negative predictive value of 84% and a positive predictive value of 97%.

Axillary UNB has a good clinical utility, based on a meta-analysis of Houssami N, Diepstraten SCE et al, in [18], on 7097 patients, with a percent of 18.4% of patients effectively referred to axillary treatment thus avoiding SNB.

4.6.2. Percutaneous biopsy procedures in locally advanced breast cancer

Locally advanced stages of the disease are usually associated with obvious ultrasound features of axillary node involvement, and ultrasound helps the biopsy of these nodes, in most cases reffering the patient to systemic preoperative treatment.

Ultrasound examination and US-guided biopsy may the only possibility to diagnose the breast cancer that presents with no identifiable breast tumor and clinically positive axillary metastasis only. When mammography is negative, biopsy of the clinically positive lymph node is the only

http://dx.doi.org/10.5772/59730

way to obtain a specimen for pathology and ultrasound could help localization and guiding the procedure.

The advantages of preoperative systemic therapy include the potential downsizing of large tumors for either conversion of inoperable disease to resectable lesions or conversion of patients to breast conservation therapy, and in vivo assessment of the response of the tumor to chemotherapy, in reference [19]. Algorithms were issued for attributing patients to preoperative systemic therapy.

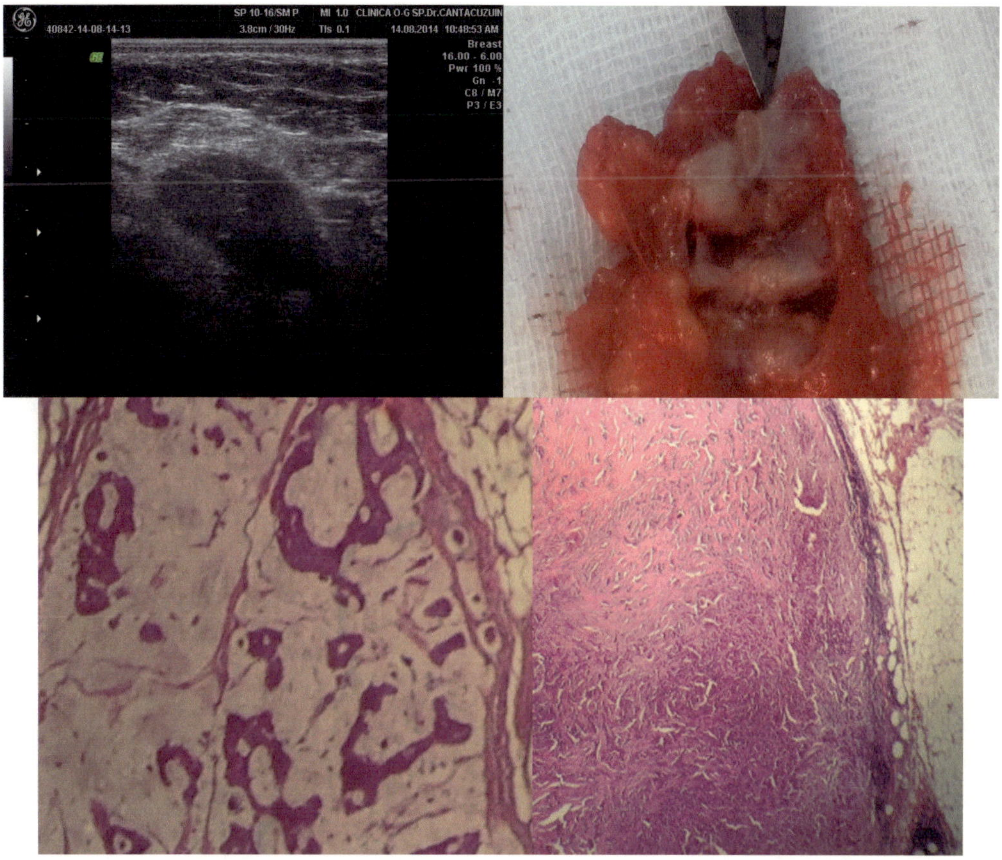

Figure 11. Patient presenting with palpable axillary lymph node. No breast tumor could be identified (mammography negative). Multiple passes were performed on the breast for core-biopsy, and the palpable node was removed by open surgery. Pathology showed axillary metastasis of invasive ductal carcinoma, with areas of mucinous carcinoma and failed to confirm the presence of the disease at the breast level.

Lee at al, in [20], consider sonographically detected axillary metastases as a clinically positive axilla, so complete ALND is recommended for patients with positive axillary biopsy, even with a clinically negative axilla, after neoadjuvant chemotherapy.

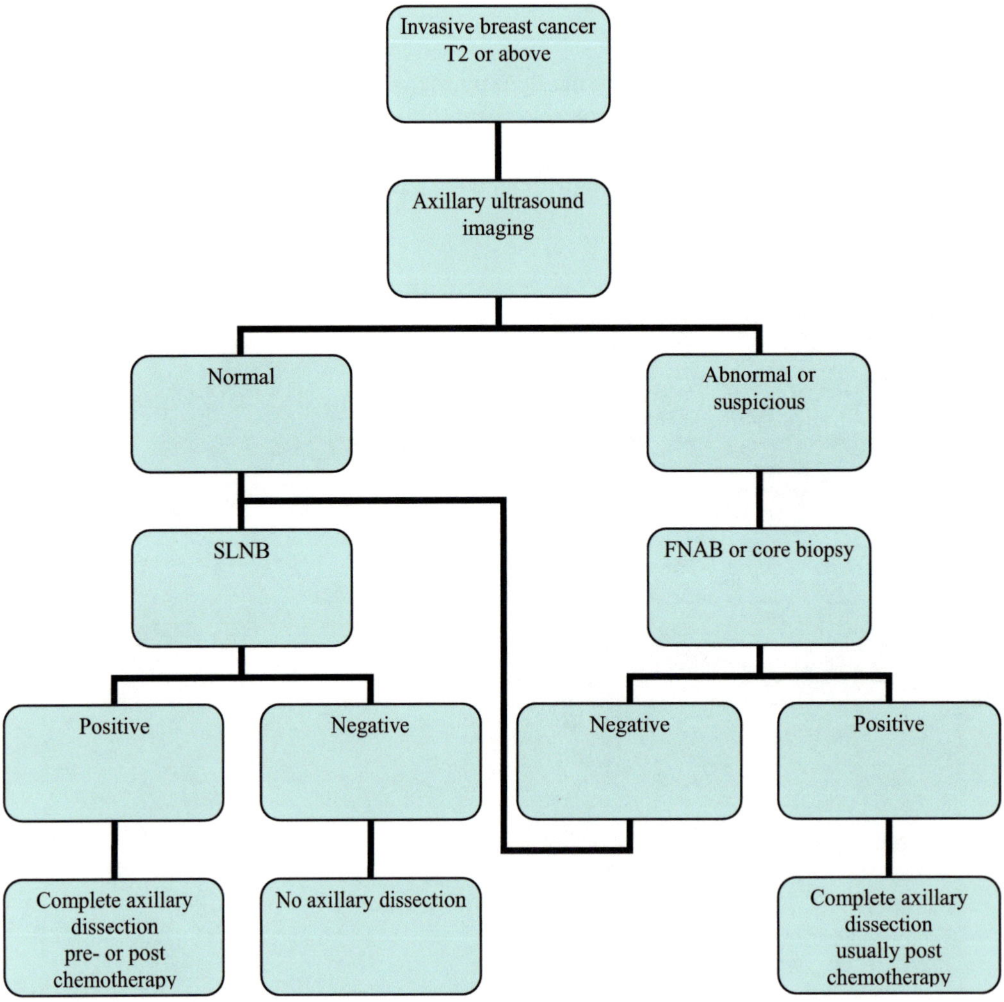

Figure 12. Algorithm for axillary assessment in patients with locally advanced invasive breast cancer (adapted from Lee MC et al, in [20]).

5. Conclusion

Axillary staging for breast cancer evolved from axillary lymph node dissection towards the lesser invasive sentinel lymph node biopsy. Nowadays, although SLNB remains the standard procedure for diagnosing axillar involvement, axillary ultrasonography is performed as the initial staging examination breast cancer patients.

In operable breast cancer, ultrasound helps identification and guide biopsy of sentinel lymph node, and/or other imaging suspicious-appearing lymph nodes. As axillary ultrasonography with either FNAB or core-biopsy is a far less invasive approach to diagnose lymph node metastasis, approximately 15 % of breast cancer patients will avoid an unnecessary SLNB and proceed directly to complete axillary dissection.

For patients with locally advanced invasive breast cancer, the recent years brought a growing practice of the routine axillary ultrasound imaging, with early referral of patients to preoperative systemic chemotherapy.

Author details

Nastasia Serban*

Address all correspondence to: serban_nastasia@yahoo.com

"Carol Davila" University of Medicine and Pharmacy, "Dr. Ion Cantacuzino"Department of Obstetrics and Gynecology, Bucharest, Romania

References

[1] Carter CL, Allen C, Henson DE. Relation of tumor size, lymph node status, and survival in 24,740 breast cancer cases. Cancer 1989;63 181-7.

[2] Whitman GJ, Lua TJ, Adejolu M, Krishnamurthy S, Sheppard D. Lymph node sonography. Ultrasound Clinics 2011;6(3) 369–380.

[3] Vassallo P, Wernecke K, Roos N, et al. Differentiation of benign from malignant superficial lymphadenopathy: the role of high-resolution US. Radiology 1992;183 215–20.

[4] Fajardo LF. Lymph nodes and cancer: a review. Frontiers of Radiation Therapy and Oncology 1994;28 1–10.

[5] Yeoh EK, Denham JW, Davies SA, Spittle MF. Primary breast cancer. Complications of axillary management. Acta Radiol Oncol 1986;25(2) 105-8.

[6] Cho N, Moon WK, Han W, Park IA, Cho J, Noh DY. Preoperative sonographic classification of axillary lymph nodes in patients with breast cancer: node-to-node correlation with surgical histology and sentinel node biopsy results. AJR American Journal of Roentgenology 2009;193 1731-7.

[7] Song SE, Seo BK, Lee SH, Yie A, Lee KY, Cho KR, Woo OH, Cha SH, Kim BH. Classification of metastatic versus non-metastatic axillary nodes in breast cancer patients: value of cortex-hilum area ratio with ultrasound. Journal of Breast Cancer 2012; 15(1) 65-70.

[8] Nastasia S, Bordea C, Russu MC, Blidaru Al, Hudita D. Axillary ultrasound and the concept of sentinel lymph node in breast cancer. Revista Societății Române de Obstetrică-Ginecologie 2008;2(LVI) 117-123.

[9] Choi JJ, Kang BJ, Kim SH, Lee JH, Jeong SH, Yim HW, Song BJ, Jung SS. Role of sonographic elastography in the differential diagnosis of axillary lymph nodes in breast cancer. Journal of Ultrasound in Medicine 2011;30(4) 429–36.

[10] Taylor K, OKeeffe S, Britton PD, Wallis MG, Treece GM, Housden J, Parashar D, Bond S, Sinnatamby R. Ultrasound elastography as an adjuvant to conventional ultrasound in the preoperative assessment of axillary lymph nodes in suspected breast cancer: a pilot study. Clinical Radiology 2011;66(11) 1064–71.

[11] Wojcinski S, Dupont J, Schmidt W, Cassel M, Hillemanns P. Real-time ultrasound elastography in 180 axillary lymph nodes: elasticity distribution in healthy lymph nodes and prediction of breast cancer metastases. BMC Medical Imaging 2012;19 12-35. Open Access. http://www.biomedcentral.com/1471-2342/12/35. DOI: 10.1186/1471-2342-12-35.

[12] Esen G, Gurses B, Yilmaz MH, Ilvan S, Ulus S, Celik V, Farahmand M, Calay OO. Gray scale and power Doppler US in the preoperative evaluation of axillary metastases in breast cancer patients with no palpable lymph nodes. European Radiology 2005;15(6) 1215–23.

[13] Moore A, Hester M, Nam MW, Brill Y M, McGrath P, Wright H, Weisinger K, Romond E, Samayoa L M. Distinct lymph nodal sonographic characteristics in breast cancer patients at high risk for axillary metastases correlate with the final axillary stage. The British Journal of Radiology 2008;81(968) 630-636.

[14] Joh JE, Han G, Kiluk JV, Laronga C, Khakpour N, Lee MC. Indications for axillary ultrasound use in breast cancer patients. Clinical Breast Cancer 2012;12 433-437.

[15] Valente SA, Levine GM, Silverstein MJ, Rayhanabad JA, Weng-Grumley JG, Ji L, Holmes DR, Sposto R, Sener SF. Accuracy of predicting axillary lymph node positivity by physical examination, mammography, ultrasonography, and magnetic resonance imaging. Annals of Surgical Oncology 2012;19(6):1825-30. DOI: 10.1245/s10434-011-2200-7.

[16] Houssami N, Ciatto S, Turner RM, Cody HS III, Macaskill P. Preoperative ultrasound-guided needle biopsy of axillary nodes in invasive breast cancer: meta-analysis of its accuracy and utility in staging the axilla. Annals of Surgery 2011;254 243-251.

[17] Holwitt DM, Swatske ME, Gillanders WE, Monsees BS, Gao F, Aft RL, Eberlein TJ, Margenthaler JA. The combination of axillary ultrasound and ultrasound-guided biopsy is an accurate predictor of axillary stage in clinically node-negative breast cancer patients. The American Journal of Surgery 2008;196 477–482.

[18] Houssami N, Diepstraten SCE, Cody H, Turner RM, Sever AM. Clinical utility of ultrasound-needle biopsy for preoperative staging of the axilla in invasive breast cancer. Anticancer Research 2014;34 1087-1098.

[19] Fisher B, Bryant J, Wolmark N, Mamounas E, Brown A, Fisher ER, Wickerham DL, Begovic M, DeCillis A, Robidoux A, Margolese RG, Cruz AB Jr, Hoehn JL, Lees AW, Dimitrov NV, Bear HD. Effect of preoperative chemotherapy on the outcome of women with operable breast cancer. Journal of Clinical Oncology 1998;16(8) 2672-2685.

[20] Lee MC, Joh JE, Chau A. Axillary staging prior to neoadjuvant chemotherapy: the roles of sentinel lymph node biopsy and axillary ultrasonography. Cancer Control 2012;4(19) 277-85.

Chapter 3

Positron Emission Mammography

Mónica Vieira Martins

Additional information is available at the end of the chapter

http://dx.doi.org/10.5772/60452

1. Introduction

1.1. Motivation

Breast cancer imaging is a good example of how medical imaging modalities can diminish the number of patients suffering from this highly prevalent and deadly disease. X-ray mammography is the most used technique for breast cancer imaging. This technique is used either as a complementary tool to clinical diagnosis or as an irreplaceable screening tool for the early detection of the disease. However, it suffers from low specificity in the detection of malignancy and low sensitivity in women with dense breast tissue. Other imaging methods such as breast Ecography and breast Magnetic Resonance Imaging play important roles as adjunct techniques to X-ray mammography. The information provided by the aforementioned techniques is, however, mainly anatomical, thus leaving space for imaging methods that are able to obtain information regarding functional or metabolic changes in tissues.

Among these, molecular imaging methods using labeled radiotracers such as Scintigraphy, SPECT, Positron Emission Tomography (PET) and PET-CT, have been found to provide useful complementary information to the anatomical methods regarding detection, diagnosis and staging of breast cancer. However, the standard technology of whole body scanners, due to its limited spatial resolution, and to its disadvantageous geometry, which limits sensitivity, have in part precluded molecular imaging using radiotracers from contributing with its full potential to the imaging of the breast.

These limitations have prompted an active interest in the development of compact positron emission tomography cameras dedicated for breast imaging, a technique named Positron Emission Mammography. In the last 20 years there has been a tremendous effort from the industry and the scientific community to develop such devices, with a variety of detector designs and geometries, innovative radiation detection schemes, new scintillation crystals and adapted image reconstruction algorithms being studied in order to optimize the technique.

Either as prototypes or as commercial equipment, PEM scanners have provided data that confirms a huge improvement in technical characteristics with regards to whole body scanner, thus showing great promise of becoming a valuable modality in the clinical practice. In fact, Positron Emission Mammography, for which there are now two commercial equipment available, has demonstrated higher detectability than PET/CT and comparable or better sensitivity than MRI. It seems now to be clear that PEM is a valuable technique when MRI cannot be used.

In this chapter we will present a review from the literature of the main equipment that have been developed for Positron Emission Mammography, emphasizing the different approaches that have been followed in the design of the scanners, the main technical outcomes and, when such information is available, the most significant results obtained in the clinical trials.

The chapter will begin with a brief description of the principles behind the tomographic method for molecular imaging of positron emission isotopes. We will then review the performance parameters and instrumentation issues more challenging in the design of dedicated PEM scanners. We will review the PEM clinical results available so far, which allow a direct comparison between PEM, PET and MRI, and which give some clues regarding the clinical utility of PEM.

2. Positron emission mammography technology

The principles underlying Positron Emission Mammography are similar to those of Positron Emission Tomography. However, since there is a requirement for high resolution and high sensitivity, specific instrumentation issues are raised during the design and development of PEM scanners. This section will begin by presenting the principles of positron emission detection for medical imaging purposes; then, the key factors regarding the technical performance of the scanner will be presented. A very brief overview on the most important issues regarding the image reconstruction will also be presented.

2.1. Positron emission and detection

Positron Emission Mammography, as well as Positron Emission Tomography, uses radiopharmaceuticals that are labeled with a positron emitting radionuclide.

The most used radiopharmaceutical for imaging cancer in PET is 18F-fluorodeoxyglucose, or ^{18}F-FDG, a glucose analogue that is labeled with the positron emitter ^{18}F. This radiotracer is used to detect glucose consumption, which is known to be increased in cancerous cells compared to normal cells. This is due to the higher metabolism of cancerous cells. The advantage of being able to image metabolism instead of anatomy, like in CT, is that the accelerated metabolic activity of cancerous cells occurs before the changes in the anatomical structures are detectable.

The tracking mechanism of 18FDG inside the cancerous cells is as follows. FDG is a glucose analog and, just like glucose, is transported into the cells by glucose transporters named

GLUT1. These transporters are known to be overexpressed in breast cancerous cells, thus contributing to increased FDG uptake [1]. Once inside the cell, FDG is phosphorylated into deoxyglucose-6-phosphate (FDG-6-PO4) by an enzyme named hexokinase. Hexokinase is also thought to be overexpressed in cancerous cells. Unlike glucose, FDG-6-PO4 does not enter further enzymatic reactions and, due to its negative charge, it remains trapped inside the cell [2]. This metabolic trapping of FDG inside the cell constitutes the basis for imaging the in vivo distribution of the tracer.

Besides ^{18}F, other radionuclides, such as ^{82}Rb, ^{15}O, ^{13}N and ^{11}C, among others, can be used to label the molecular probes used in PET.

Once emitted from the radiopharmaceutical, the positron travels a given amount of space in matter, while dissipating its kinetic energy through interactions with electrons and surrounding nuclei. At the end of its path, the positron combines with an electron in its vicinity, in an annihilation reaction whereby the total mass of the electron and the positron is converted into high energy photons. The rest-mass energy of both positron and electron is 511 keV. If both particles are at rest at the time of annihilation, the two resulting 511 keV photons will be emitted in opposite directions.

The gamma rays thus emitted can interact with the tissues of the patient either by photoelectric effect or by Compton scatter. Both photon attenuation and scatter result in image degradation since, in the first case, emission counts are lost and, in the second, the measured spatial information is inaccurate. Whereas the correction for the effect of attenuation is fairly simple if a transmission scan is available, the correction for the scatter effect not as straightforward.

If the photons are not absorbed by the matter in the patient body, they can be detected externally in coincidence by using opposed pairs of scintillator crystals. Each luminous signal produced in the crystals is transformed into an electrical signal. A coincidence event happens when such two electrical signals are registered in a coincidence electronic circuit within a time frame that is defined by a coincidence time window.

The imaginary line that unites the two activated crystals in a coincidence event is called a line of response (LOR). The number of counts that are detected along the several LORs during an exam is stored in an histogram and used for image reconstruction purposes. Alternatively, list mode format can be used. In list mode format, the relevant information regarding the event, such as the activated crystals, the deposited energy and a time stamp, is stored sequentially on disk and used directly for image reconstruction.

2.2. The performance of a scanner

Of main importance for the performance of a PET scanner are its photon sensitivity and its spatial, energy and temporal resolutions. The geometry, the detector crystals and the electronics of the system all impact on the above. In this paragraph we will overview the main aspects that affect these parameters, highlighting the most common differences between traditional clinical scanners and high resolution scanners.

The **photon sensitivity** is defined as the fraction of 511 keV photon pairs emitted from the imaging subject that are detected by the imaging system [3]. It is important that a scanner has the higher photon sensitivity possible since a higher fraction of detected photons will impact on better statistics of the acquired data and, consequently, on lower noise level of the final reconstructed images. The photon sensitivity in a clinical PET system is low. In dedicated or high resolution scanners, The sensitivity is usually improved by increasing the scanner geometric efficiency, that is, the probability that the emitted photon transverses the detected material, or by increasing the intrinsic detector efficiency.

Usually, the scanner geometric efficiency is enhanced in dedicated scanners relatively to traditional scanners mainly because the detector is brought closer to the imaging subject.

The geometric efficiency can also be increased by packing the detector elements as tightly as possible and by covering the region to be imaged with as much detector as possible. The other aspect that influences the scanner photon sensitivity is the intrinsic detector efficiency. This is defined as the likelihood that photons transversing the detector material will be stopped [3]. It depends mainly on the scintillator crystals that are used as detector elements. Scintillator crystals that have high density (ϱ), with high effective atomic number (Z_{eff}) have maximum ability to stop the 511 keV photons. In fact, a high density crystal favors the photon interaction and a high effective atomic number maximizes the probability of photoelectric interactions within the crystal, with respect to Compton events. The quantity that maximizes the crystal stopping power is $\varrho . Z_{eff}^5$. A scintillator that has a high stopping power will have a short attenuation length.

Table 1 lists the values of Z_{eff}, ϱ, the attenuation length and some other properties of the most common scintillator crystals used in PET scanners. The decay time determines the time resolution of the scanner and the light output determines the detector energy resolution and has effects also in the image resolution. Both these parameters will be discussed later.

Sodium iodide doped with thallium (NaI(Tl)) was the detector initially used in PET scanners. It has a very high light output (38 photons/keV), resulting in good energy and spatial resolutions [4]. However, its slow decay time leads to increased detector dead time and a high random coincidence rate (see below the discussion for system time resolution). Its low density results in a low stopping power (high attenuation length) when compared to the other crystals used in PET. Sodium iodine was first replaced by BGO (bismuth germanate: $Bi_4Ge_3O_{12}$) that, despite its high decay time and poor light output, has an excellent stopping power.

More recently, other crystals that combine better light output with high stopping power have been introduced to PET. LSO (lutetium oxyorthosilicate: Lu2SiO5) has a high stopping power and a good light yield but, due to intrinsic properties of the crystal, its overall resolution is not as good as NaI(Tl) [5]. GSO (gadolinium orthosilicate: Gd_2SiO_5), despite its lower stopping power and light output, has better energy resolution than LSO. Both crystals are in use in PET scanners.

The **spatial resolution** describes the ability of the system to distinguish two closely spaced point sources. In PET, the fundamental limit of spatial resolution is imposed by the nature of positron annihilation. In fact, the emitted positron describes, before annihilating, a given path of variable length and direction. Therefore, the detected LOR contains the positron annihilation

http://dx.doi.org/10.5772/60452

	Effective Z	Density (g/cm^3)	Attenuation length (mm)	Relative light output (% NaI)	Decay time (ns)
Sodium Iodide	51	3.7	29.1	100	230
BGO	75	7.2	10.4	15	300
LSO	66	7.4	11.4	75	42
GSO	59	6.7	14.1	20	60
LYSO	65	7.1	1.2	107	40
LuAP	65	8.3	*	30	17
LuYAP	60	7.1	*	34	23

Table 1. Properties of common scintillator crystals used in positron emission tomography.Adapted from [3] and from [6] (LuAP and LuYAP data). * Data not found.

point, not the positron emission point, and these two points can be several millimeters apart. This positron range effect degrades the spatial resolution of the images. (Figure 1a). The positron range depends upon the energy of the emitted positron and upon the electronic density of the medium. It has been estimated a value of 0.22 mm FWHM for the positron range emitted from ^{18}F in water, the major component of human cells [7].

In addition to the positron range, the acollinearity effect also leads to resolution degradation in PET systems. This effect is caused by the fact that the annihilation photons are almost never anti-parallel, since usually the positron and the electron are not exactly at rest when they annihilate. As a consequence, the detected line of response does not contain the point of positron-electron annihilation (Figure 1b). The degradation of the spatial resolution due to the accolinearity effect worsens as the detector diameter increases.

Another significant factor that limits PET spatial resolution is the size of the detector element. Spatial resolution may be improved significantly by reducing the detector pixel size. This is especially important in small diameter or dedicated PET scanners, where the pixel size dominates image resolution over the non-collinearity effect, which is minor for small detector diameters. Typical clinical systems use 4.0–6.0 mm detector pixel sizes, whereas small animal use detector pixels of 1.5–2.0 mm and positron emission mammography scanners use pixel sizes of 1.8–3.0 mm.

A final important factor that affects PET spatial resolution is the parallax error. This error occurs when the crystal depth at which the photon interaction takes place, known as Depth of Interaction (DOI), is not known. In this case, the LOR that unites the two activated crystals does not necessarily contain the true LOR (Figure 1c). For photons entering the scintillators at oblique angles there will be a mismatch between the true and the measured line of response. This degrading effect has greater impact in scanners where the distance between opposed detectors is smaller, like dedicated cameras. Good spatial resolution is of crucial importance for these cameras.

To improve photon sensitivity, the scintillator crystals that compose these dedicated scanners are usually long crystals. Therefore, not surprisingly, the ability to obtain DOI information has become an important factor in the design of high resolution PET scanners [8], with different strategies being followed to perform such measurements.

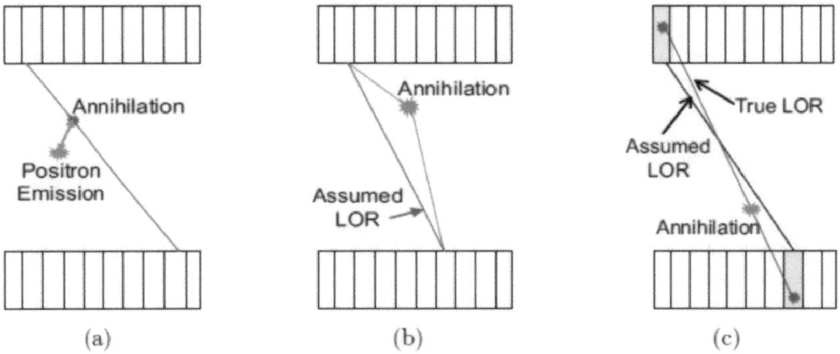

Figure 1. Schematic drawings of some of the effects that degrade spatial resolution in PET: a) the positron range, b) the accolinearity effect and c) the Depth of Interaction effect or parallax error.

The **energy resolution** indicates the precision with which the system can measure the incoming photon energy. A good energy resolution is important because it allows the use of a narrow energy window without significantly compromising photon sensitivity.

A narrow energy window helps to prevent contamination from photons that undergo scatter before interacting with the scintillator crystal, since the scatter process implies the loss of energy. It may also help to reduce the rate of random photon events, since a part of these photons undergo scatter. Random, or accidental, coincidences, occur when photons proceeding from different annihilations are detected within a same timing window and, although spatially uncorrelated, its detection is considered as a valid coincidence.

Energy resolution may be improved by using crystals with hight scintillation light output. A typical value for clinical PET scanners energy resolution is 25% FWHM at 511 keV [3].

The **time resolution** determines how well the system can decide whether two incoming photons arrived simultaneously. Good time resolution allows the use of a narrow time window, thus reducing random event's detection without compromising photon sensitivity. The reducing of random events is also important as it helps to prevent the system from saturating in high count statistics studies. The parameter that most strongly determines the temporal coincidence timing window is the scintillator decay time: a fast scintillator allows the selection of a narrow time window. A typical value for clinical PET scanners time resolution is 3 ns FWHM at 511 keV [3].

The scintillation light from the crystals is read from **photodetectors**. In PET, are most commonly either photomultiplier tubes (PMT) or semiconductor based photodiodes. Photomultiplier tubes are the oldest and most reliable technology to detect and measure low levels of scintillation light. They have a high gain in the photoelectric conversion, which leads to high signal-to-noise ratios. Besides simple PMT's, a class of PMTs has been developed that provides not only energy information but also spatial information about the detected light. These PMTs, named Position-Sensitive PMTs (PS-PMT) have been found to be useful in the design of high resolution PET scanners [9].

PMTs have two major drawbacks. They have low quantum efficiency, meaning that the ratio between the incident photons and the primary produced electrons is low. In addition, PMTs are big devices, often with a small field of view, and this may constitute a drawback, especially when they are to be used in small dedicated scanners. In recent years there has also been great progress in the development of semiconductor photodetector arrays. These can be the PIN photodiode, the avalanche photodiode (APD) and the silicon drift detector (SDD). Among these, the APDs are the most used in PET cameras. Semiconductor photodetectors have many advantages over PMTs: they are very compact; they are insensitive to magnetic fields, which makes them good candidates for PET-MRI devices; they are available with large active areas; they have a very high efficiency [10]. The main disadvantages of APDs are their sensitivity to temperature and bias voltage.

2.3. Image reconstrucion

For many years, the problem of reconstructing an image from the projection data acquired in Positron Emission Tomography was addressed with analytic approaches which were inherited from X-ray computed tomography. Analytic algorithms such as filtered backprojection (FBP) are based on the direct inversion of the Radon transform. They are fast, linear, predictable, and their properties are very well known. The inversion of the Radon transform is derived for a continuous sampling and discretized afterward for sampled data [99]. Analytic algorithms are based on an idealized mathematical model for the data, the linear integral model, according to which the number of coincidence photon pairs detected along a LOR is approximately linearly proportional to the integral of the tracer density along a LOR. This model over-simplifies the physics inherent to the emission and detection processes in PET, limiting the accuracy of the images reconstructed with analytical algorithms.

In alternative to the analytic image reconstruction algorithms, model based algorithms, which can include accurate physical and statistical models of the systems, can be used. In opposition to analytical algorithms, they incorporate the discreteness of the data from the beginning. Their use usually results in improved image accuracy. As their formulation results frequently in large sets of nonlinear equations that must be solved by iterative methods, this class of algorithms is usually referred to as iterative image reconstruction algorithms. Furthermore, if statistical functions are used to derive them, they are said to be statistical iterative reconstruction algorithms. The use of iterative methods based on probability models for image reconstruction was already effective in the field of astronomy in the early 1970's (Lucy, 1974, Richardson 1972). Later, in 1976, Rockmore and Macovsky introduced the Maximum Likelihood approach in the field of medical imaging. The Ordered Subsets – Expectation Maximization (OSEM) algorithm was proposed in 1994 by Hudson and Larkin as an accelerated version of the ML-EM method and has since gained wide acceptance as a standard reconstruction method in PET. Nowadays, the most used algorithms for image reconstruction in PET belong to the class of iterative statistical algorithms.

3. Positron emission mammography scanners

A design of a dedicated positron emission imaging system for breast cancer was first presented in 1994 as a feasibility study for a positron emission mammography unit. Since then, more than ten other systems have been developed, two of which have become commercially available [11, 12]. Those systems differ in the number, geometry and mobility of the detectors used, with consequences on the patient positioning; its ability or not to perform biopsy; the different radiation detection scheme used, including different scintillation crystals; on the strategies used for image reconstruction from the measured projections. In this section we will review the instrumentation issues that impact on the performance of the equipment that use positron emission mammography to image disease. We will emphasize on the most demanding aspects of these dedicated instruments, showing why they hold the promise for an improved early detection of disease.

3.1. The PEM-I system

A design of a dedicated positron emission imaging system for breast cancer was first presented in 1994 by Thompson [13] from the Montreal Neurological Institute of the McGill University, Canada, as a feasibility study for a positron emission mammography unit.

The developed scanner was designed to fit a mammographic unit, so that conventional mammograms could also be performed in the same gantry, thus allowing exact registration of the emission and of the conventional mammographic images [14]. For such purposes, the system included a co-registration tool to facilitate registration between radiographic and metabolic images [15]. A schematic diagram of the scanner is presented in Figure 2.

The developed scanner consists on two planar 2x2 detector arrays of blocks of bismuth germanate (BGO) crystals placed above and below the compressed breast. The detector blocks measure 36x36x20 mm^3 and are segmented into 1.9x1.9 mm^2 pixels [16]. The separation between the detector heads can be adjusted to match the thickness of the breast. The system uses position sensitive photomultiplier tubes (PS-PMT) that are optically coupled to the crystal blocks. Although the PS-PMTs cover a surface of 72x72 mm^2, their useful field-of-view (FOV) is only of 65x55 mm^2. The coordinates of the coincidence on opposing PS-PMT faces are decoded by the system electronics and corrected for spatial distortion and efficiency [17].

The images from this system are obtained by performing a limited-angle weighted-backprojection algorithm. This consists on dividing the image into several equidistant planes and backprojecting the lines or response (LOR) onto those planes. With this technique, the image plane closest to the site of the tumor has the most focused image, while all the other planes present more blurred images, as it can be seen in the schematic diagram of Figure 3. This is known as the focal plane effect. The reconstruction scheme is said to be 'weighted backprojection' because the values that are added to a given plane in the image matrix are weighted accordingly to the probability of detection of an annihilation in that plane, the crystals efficiencies and the photon attenuation along the path to the crystal [14].

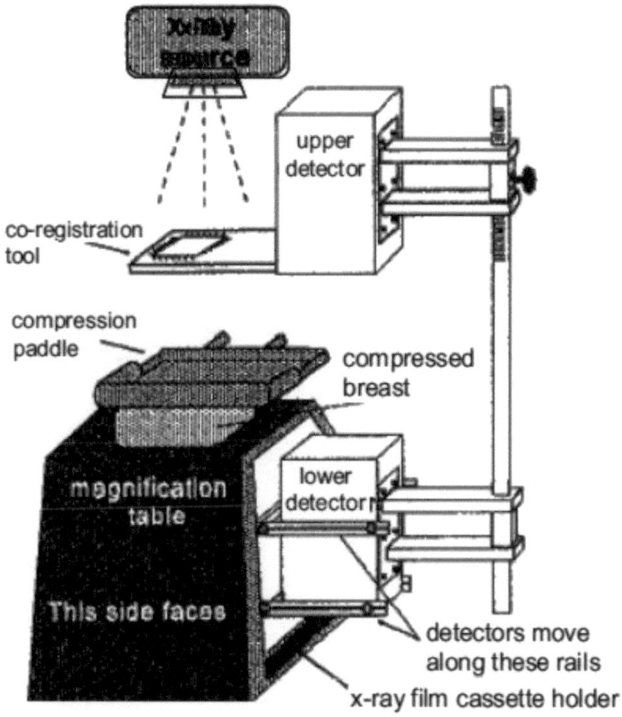

Figure 2. Schematic drawing of the PEM-I detector plates (white areas) mounted on a conventional mammographic unit (gray areas). From [15].

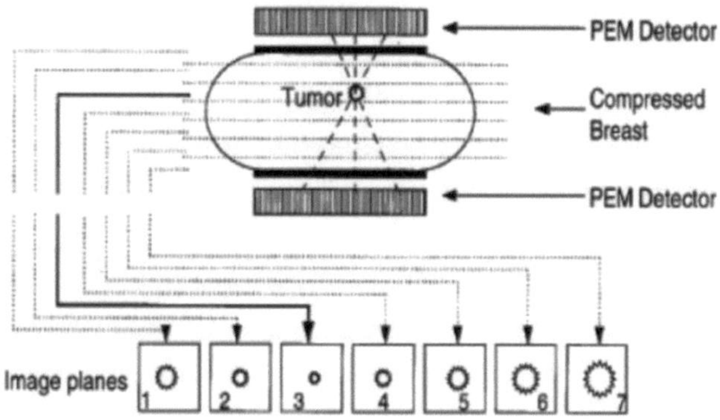

Figure 3. Weighted backprojection used in the PEM-I scanner. From [18].

The complete system has a spatial resolution of 2.8 mm FWHM, a time resolution of 12 ns and an efficiency of 3% at a detector separation of 55 mm [19]. It is estimated that the system is not able to detect tumors with a tumor-to-background ratio lower than 6:1 [20].

The preliminary clinical trials, performed with 16 subjects, reported 80% sensitivity and 100% specificity. The accuracy of the exam, computed as the ratio of the sum of the true findings (positive and negative) to the total number of lesions, was 86% [18]. For mammography exams performed on the same subjects, those values were, respectively, 90%, 50% and 81%. The smallest cancerous lesion detected with PEM-I was 1.1x1.1x0.9 cm^3. The lower value of sensitivity with PEM, with respect to mammography, was due, according to the authors, to the small FOV of the PEM device and to the impossibility of imaging tumors localized close to the chest wall (less than 2 cm). These limitations are related to the PMTs used, whose useful field of view is significantly smaller than its area, preventing imaging near their edges. Figure 4 shows a typical set of images obtained with PEM-I, each image corresponding to a plane of the sample, with a visible site of FDG uptake in a region close to the chest wall [19].

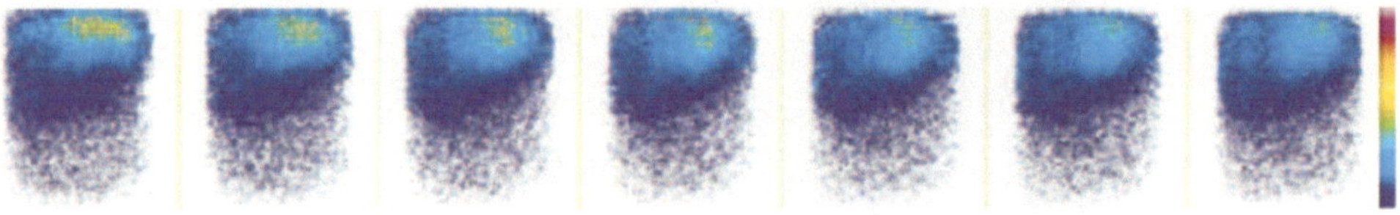

Figure 4. A typical set of images obtained with the PEM-I scanner. Each image corresponds to a plane, with the left-most image corresponding to the image plane closer to the upper detector. A visible site of FDG uptake can be seen in a region close to the chest wall. From [19].

3.2. The Naviscan PEM system

The original idea of Thompson for a PEM system was further developed by Weinberg and colleagues, for the Naviscan PET System. The Naviscan PEM Flex consists of two 5.6×17.3 cm^2 opposed detector heads [21] that can be fit on a steriotactic mammography unit [22]. This way, emission and transmission scans can be obtained. Data acquisition is performed by moving the detectors along a linear path, in order to image as much breast as possible. The PEM detectors translation allows to image an area equal to the entire X-ray field of view [23]. The system can also work separately from the mammography unit, allowing closer chest wall access. Figure 5 shows the PEM Flex system mounted in a stereotactic X-ray mammography unit.

Each detector head contains twelve 13×13 crystal blocks, each coupled to a compact PS-PMT. The crystals are 2×2×10 mm^3 of a mixed-lutetium silicate [21].

For each segment of the scan, list mode data are acquired, histogrammed and reconstructed by backprojection. This allows the operator to view partial images during the scan acquisition. At the end of the entire scan, the complete list mode data are reconstructed using a maximum-likelihood expectation-maximization algorithm.

The intrinsic spatial resolution of the system is 1.5 mm FHWM [23]. The image resolution is 2.5 mm FWHM in the plane perpendicular to the displacement and 6 mm between planes. Energy resolution was measured as 14% for 511 keV. The timing window used was 9 ns.

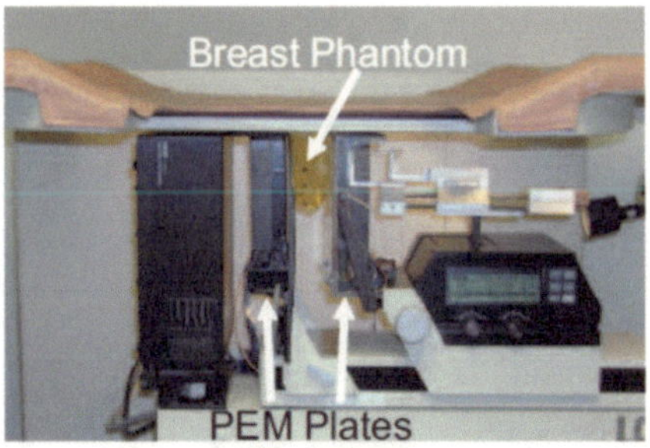

Figure 5. The PEM Flex system mounted in a stereotactic X-ray mammography unit. From [22].

The clinical trials performed so far [24, 25] were all performed on patients with known breast cancer or suspected lesions. Hence, they provide little information on the specificity of the technique. In one of these studies [25], PEM was able to visualize 39 out of 44 lesions. The non visualized lesions ranged in size from a 1 mm ductal carcinoma in situ (DCIS) to a 1 cm infiltrating ductal carcinoma. Some lesions could not be visualized due to limitations on how posterior the breast tissue is observable by the device. Others, as interpreted by the authors of the study, due to the variability in the metabolic activity of breast cancer cells, similarly to what happens with whole body PET.

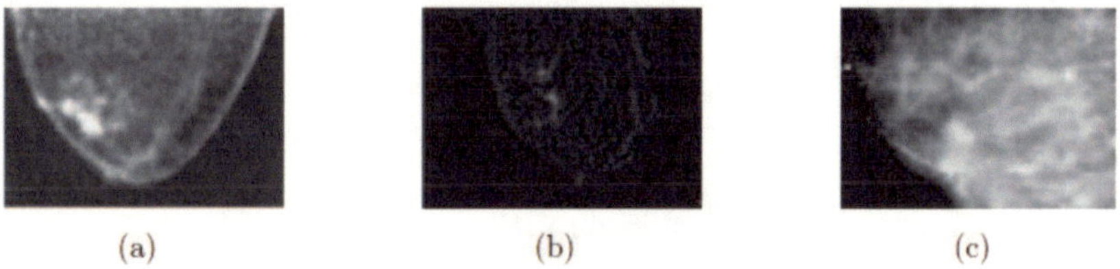

Figure 6. Image of DCIS obtained with the PEM Flex scanner a), with MRI b) and with mammography c). Neither MRI nor mammography could detect the DCIS lesion seen in the PEM image. From [25].

The most encouraging finding in this trial was the fact that PEM was able to visualize DCIS not visualized by mammography, breast ecography or MRI. An example of such a case can be seen in Figure 6. The smallest lesion detected by PEM in this study was a 2 mm duct of DCIS. This preliminary clinical trial seems to indicate that the technology is promising and worthy of further investigation.

3.3. The West Virginia University — Jefferson Lab PEM system

Another PEM system was developed and tested at the West Virginia University and at the Jefferson Laboratory by Raylman and colleagues [26]. This PEM system, which is mounted on a stereotactic biopsy table, consists of two square 10×10 cm^2 detector arrays of discrete 3×3×10 mm^3 GSO crystals. The scintillation light is collected by arrays of PS-PMTs. An image of the scanner mounted on the biopsy table, together with a torso phantom can be seen in Figure 7.

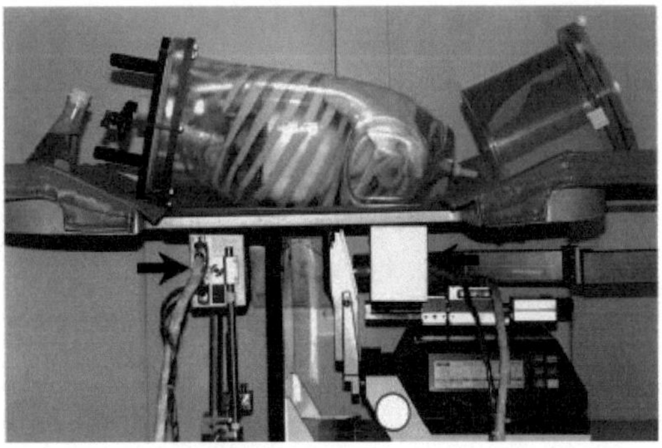

Figure 7. Image of the West Virginia University - Jefferson Laboratory PEM system. The PEM detector heads, mounted in a biopsy table, are highlighted by the black arrows. A torso phantom can be seen in the table. From [27].

Since one of the goals of the system is to perform PEM guided biopsies, a trigonometric algorithm was developed to determine the lesion stereotactic coordinates. This algorithm uses two PEM images that are acquired at two symmetric angles (±15○).

PEM images acquired in a single detector position were initially reconstructed using a weighted backprojection algorithm similar to the used for the PEM-I system described above, or by a limited angle tomography scheme [23]. Later, the use of acquired data at two detector positions (±15○) [28] to guide stereotactic biopsy motivated the use of an adapted Maximum Likelihood - Expectation Maximization algorithm.

The described acquisition scenario was compared with multiple acquisitions between the same limiting angles, at small uniform increments [29]. The results were somehow mixed, with no clear evidence of significant advantage of one acquisition scenario over the other, although less artifacts were observed with the multiple angle acquisition.

This lead to a study of the complete angular sampling around the breast [30] through step and shoot acquisitions. Not surprisingly, this study showed that the complete angular sampling provided better image quality with respect to a single acquisition with stationary detectors. The study also revealed some of the weaknesses of the system, such as the low rate acquisition capability and the lack of DOI information.

Posterior work reports a new design of the scanner, now named PEM-PET [31], as it means to be a tomographic system. This system has four planar detector heads that can rotate around the breast. The detector crystal used is now LYSO, with 2×2×15 mm^3 individual detector elements. The PEM-PET system has 2 mm FHWM resolution, possessing, as its anterior version, the ability to guide biopsy. The initial clinical studies have shown the ability of the system to detect lesions also detected by standard methods [32].

3.4. The Duke University — Jefferson Lab PEM system

Another system was developed at the Jefferson Laboratory and Duke University to image the compressed breast [33]. This PEM system has two opposed planar 15×20 cm^2 detectors that

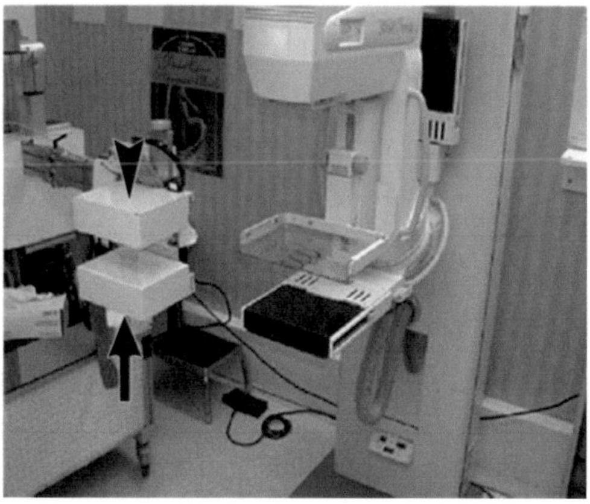

Figure 8. Image of the Duke University - Jefferson Laboratory PEMsystem positioned in a mammography unit. The PEM detectors are highlighted by black arrows.From [34].

acquire data without rotational or translational movements. The detector arrays are composed of 3×3×10 mm^3 of lutetium gadolinium oxyorthosilicate, LGSO. The scintillation light is collected by arrays of PS-PMTs. This system is used mounted on an X-ray mammography unit, although the PEM detector heads must be removed to acquire the X-ray image. The distance between the detector heads can be adjusted to match the size of the breast. Image reconstruction is performed by means of the backprojection scheme. The image spatial resolution varied from 4.8 mm to 6 mm, depending on the acceptance angles of the lines of response. An image of the system can be seen in Figure 8.

A pilot clinical trial was performed using this system [34]. This trial included 23 patients with suspected breast malignancies. Therefore, it does not provide meaningful information concerning the specificity of the technique. In this study, where the majority of the evaluated lesions had diameters smaller than 2.5 cm, PEM presented a sensitivity of 86%. The size of the three malignant lesions that PEM was unable to detect varied from 8 mm to 15 mm. The system was able to detect a 4 mm DCIS that was not detected by mammography.

3.5. The maxPET system

A dedicated PET camera for mammary and axillary region imaging, maxPET, was designed and constructed at the Crump Institute for Biological Imaging [35]. This group used an alternative scheme to couple the crystal arrays to the PMT's, in order to avoid the problems associated with the inactive area near the PMT edges. The maxPET system consisted of two 15×15 cm^2 planar scintillation detector plates, each composed of several modular detectors. The detectors are composed of arrays of 3×3×20 mm^3 LSO crystals, each crystal array being coupled to an optical fiber which in turn is coupled to a PS-PMT. The use of the optical fiber allows the exact match between the crystal area and the active PMT dimensions, thus avoiding gaps between detector modules. It also provides better imaging close to the chest wall, since the plates are active out to the edge of the field-of-view. The main disadvantage of the fiber-optic coupling is the loss of scintillation light.

The two detector plates can be mounted in a gantry allowing variable plates separation, detector plates rotation and angular motion. Based on Monte Carlo simulation, the expected intrinsic spatial resolution of the scanner was about 2.3 mm [36]. A prototype of this system was assembled but, to our knowledge, no clinical test were ever performed.

A second prototype of this detector was build, with modified geometry and electronics. The integration of this system with a dedicated CT system was exploited [37].

3.6. The LBNL PEM system

The PEM scanner developed at the Lawrence Berkeley National Laboratory (LBNL) has two major differences from the PEM scanners described here: it has a rectangular geometry, with four detector plates surrounding the breast and it has Depth of Interaction measurements capabilities [38].

The system uses a 6 ns time window and has 5% sensitivity at the center of the FOV. The measured spatial resolution of the scanner is almost uniform in the entire field-of-view, ranging from 1.9 mm FWHM at the FOV centre to 2.1 mm at the FOV corner [38]. Images of a mini-Derenzo phantom show that the smallest lesion resolved by the system is 2.4 mm in diameter.

In the context of the development of this scanner, a simulation study was done to compare the presented rectangular detector configuration with a dual stationary detector system, such as some of the systems presented above. For such purpose it was used the Fisher information matrix, an analytical computation that allows to characterize how easily a change of one parameter in the source distribution can be identified from the measured data [40]. This study has shown that the rectangular system with Depth of Interaction capability has a higher signal-to-noise ratio for detection tasks and a lower bias at a given noise level for quantitation tasks. It is worth stressing that this study did not include the case of a rotating dual head scanner [39]. The LBNL PEM system consists of four detector plates that cover a rectangular 8.2×6.0×5.0 cm^3 field of view. The detector modules contain arrays of 3×3×30 mm^3 LSO crystals that are coupled to a single photomultiplier tube (PMT) in one end and to a photodiode array (PD) on the other end. The ratio between the signals of the PMT and the PD allow the estimation of the Depth of Interaction of the photon [41]. The achieved DOI resolution ranges from 6 mm FWHM at the PD end to 11 mm FWHM at the PMT end [42].

The image reconstruction task for this scanner has been subject of an intense work. In an initial stage, image reconstruction was performed with a filtered backprojection based reconstruction algorithm that took into account the existence of DOI information and the irregular angular sampling of the scanner [43, 44]. Later, a list mode penalized maximum likelihood algorithm using Gaussian priors was developed [40, 45, 46]. A Monte Carlo based scatter correction algorithm was also developed [46]. To our knowledge, this scanner has never been tested with clinical data.

3.7. The YAP-PEM system

The YAP-PEM prototype was developed within a collaboration of the Italian Universities of Pisa, Ferrara, Bologna and Roma [47]. The technology of this device derives from a small animal scanner previously developed by the group. The YAP-PEM scanner has been designed with the aim of detecting 5 mm breast lesions in diameter and an activity ratio of 10:1 between the cancer and the breast tissue. The device is composed of two stationary detector heads made of yttrium aluminium perovskite (YAlO3) scintillators doped with cerium (YAP:Ce). This is a scintillator crystal that produces a light output of about 20 photons/keV, has a decay constant of 30 ns and a density of 5.4 g/cm^3 [48]. It has, however, a low Z number. Each detector head has a detection area of 6×6 cm^2 that comprises 30×30 detection elements with 2×2×30 mm^3 each. The system uses PS-PMTs to collect the scintillation light. The distance between the detectors can range from 5 to 10 cm, depending on the breast compression used.

For image reconstruction purposes, the ML-EM algorithm has been adapted to the planar nature of the acquired data, in order to obtain a pseudo-tomographic imaging method [49]. This method works on data that is converted into histograms that are indicated for planar data. These are known as planograms [50]. Geometrical symmetries are used to speed up the computations.

Monte Carlo simulation and image reconstruction studies performed for the YAP-PEM scanner indicate that the scanner is expected to have capability of discriminating 5 mm tumors in a target-to-background ratio of 10:1. However, due to the planar nature of the data, if two sources lie on the same axial plane, the system cannot discriminate them, as it can be seen in Figure 10.

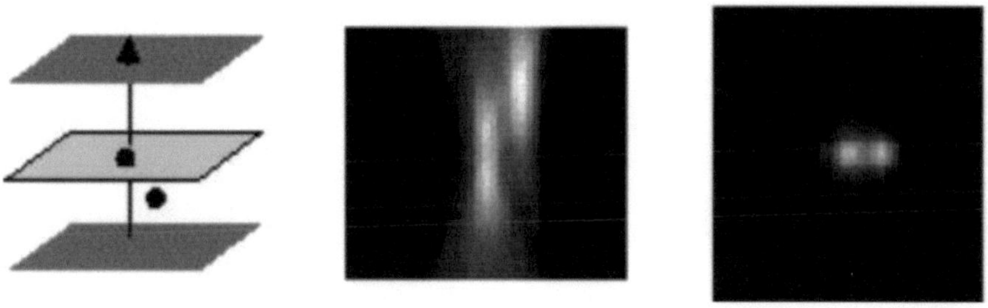

Figure 9. Phantom images obtained with the YAP-PEM prototype. Due to the planar nature of the scanner's data, if two sources lie on a same axial plane, the system cannot discriminate them. From [49].

3.8. The Clear-PEM system

The Clear-PEM system was developed within the framework of the CrystalClear collaboration, in CERN. The system, which was designed to allow the examination of the breast and the axilla regions, is composed of a dual-plate detector head that is housed in a robotic mechanical gantry, as represented in Figure 11. For the breast examination, the patient lays in the prone position with the breast hanging through an aperture in the patient. The two detector heads are positioned in each side of the breast, as represented in Figure 11, and the projection data are acquired at several angular positions. The detector heads can be positioned at different separation distances, allowing for the accommodation of different breast sizes.

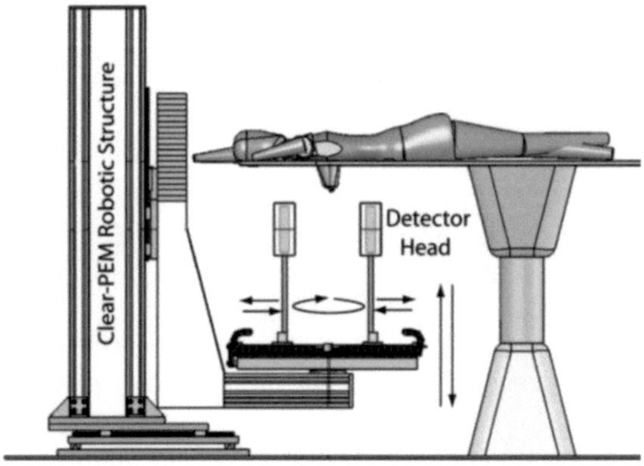

Figure 10. Representation of the Clear-PEM system.From [51].

The detector heads cover a 16.2×14.1 cm^2 FoV. Each detector head holds 96 detector modules, is constituted of a total of 3072 LYSO:Ce crystals, each crystal having 2×2×20 mm^3. A scheme of a detector head is shown in Figure 12a. The distribution of the crystals within, the detector plates is as follows. Each detector plate is constituted of a set of four structures named supermodules, each one with 14×4 cm^2, placed side by side. Each supermodule is composed of 12×2 modules that, in turn, are composed of an array of 4×8 LYSO:Ce crystals. Therefore, each detector plate is constituted of 48×64 LYSO:Ce crystals.

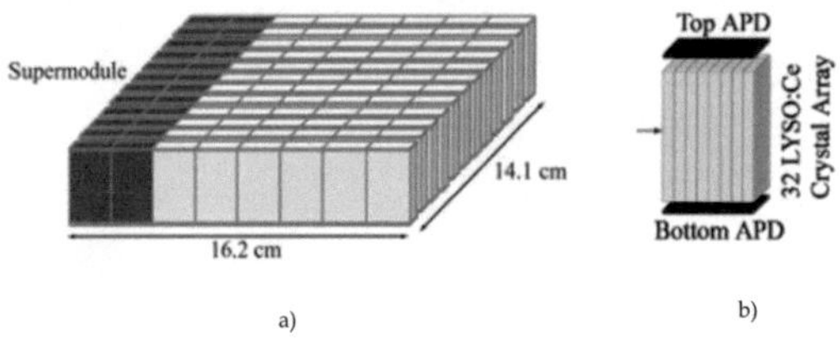

Figure 11. Clear-PEM detectors. a) Representation of a Clear-PEM detector head, with an highlighted detector supermodule. From [51]. b) Representation of a Clear-PEM detector module with the double readout scheme. From [52].

The readout of each module is performed by two 32-pixel avalanche photodiodes that are optically coupled to each side of the module, as shown in Figure 12b. This double readout scheme allows the DOI measurement. The DOI coordinate within the crystal is estimated from the asymmetry of the collected light at the top and bottom APD pixels. Experimental results have shown that, with this scheme, it is possible to obtain a 2 mm FWHM DOI resolution [53]. This measurement is important since it increases the uniformity all over the field-of-view of the scanner. This feature is not common in the universe of the positron emission mammography dedicated scanners and therefore it is perhaps one of the most important characteristics of this scanner. The processing of the detector analogical signals, including the readout, the low noise amplification, the sampling and the storage are implemented in dedicated ASICs (Application Specific Integrated Circuits) integrated in the detection plates. The output analogue sampled pulses are digitized by Analogue Digital Converters (ADC) and transmitted to the data acquisitions system (DAQ). This system, based on FPGA (Field Programmable Gate Arrays), is responsible for the data reduction and storage. Data is send from here to a trigger system that selects two-photon events in coincidence within a programmable timing window and, at each trigger, the relevant data frames are send to the acquisition PC where energy and time information are analyzed [54]. For events with more than one active crystal in a detector head, due to Compton scattering, an event reconstruction position algorithms is used to assign the coordinates of the interaction. Those events that are within the selected energy window are validated, their final coordinates being used to define the LORs that are stored in a list-mode file [53]. Images are reconstructed using 3D statistical iterative algorithms or 2D algebraic techniques [55–57]. Phantom studies showed that the scanner is suitable for milimetric tumor detection; Derenzo phantom studies showed that lesions up to 2 mm in diameter can be clearly seen; a gelatin breast phantom indicated that lesions up to 3 mm in diameter can be detected. The first prototype, installed at the Institute of Nuclear Sciences Applied to Health, Coimbra, Portugal, was used for the first tests in a preclinical environment [58].

More recently, the ClearPEM scanner has been used to create a multimodal PEM and ultrasound scanner [59]. The aim of this system is to provide high resolution, high sensitivity and high specificity metabolic information from PEM matched with 3D high resolution anatomic information. The new ClearPEM-Sonic scanner also provides elastographic information from ultrasound, further improving the specificity of the multimodality scanner. This second prototype is installed at the Hôpital Nord, in Marseille, France, and has confirmed a spatial resolution of about 1.5 mm in phantom studies. The system allows the co-registration of US/ClearPEM and elastography/ClearPEM with an alignment precision of about 2 mm. The first clinical trial has confirm the ability to detect very small lesions only seen by MRI, although lesions very close to the chest wall are left undetected [60].

3.9. The MAMMI system

MAMMI (MAMmography with Molecular Imaging) is a dedicated breast PET, commercialized by Oncovision, which has certification in Europe and has recently received FDA approval [61].

Instead of the more often used small pixelated crystal arrays, this scanner uses continuous LYSO crystals coupled to PSPMTs.

The MAMMI prototype is a full ring PET consisting on 12 detector modules forming a dodecagon with a scanner aperture of 186 mm [12]. Each detector module uses 10 mm thick scintillation crystals with 40x40mm^2 face. The back face of the crystals are coupled to the PS-PMTs. The detector has a 18% energy resolution at 511 keV, an intrinsic resolution of 1.6 mm and a DOI resolution of 4 mm.

The system aperture provides a 170 mm diameter FoV. The coincidences are allowed between a detector module and its seven opposite modules, providing a transaxial FoV aperture of 170 mm diameter. The axial FoV length is 40 mm per frame; an elevator allows the sequential move of the ring detector in step and shoot mode to increase the axial FoV to 170 mm. A timing window of 5 ns is used.

During image reconstruction the crystal faces are discretized into 2x2 mm^2 pixels. Images are reconstructed with standard 3D ML-EM with a voxel size of 1x1x1 mm^3. The system matrix was obtained through calculation of the solid angle of every voxel with respect to the detection surface. Image reconstruction takes into account dead time, scatter and random events correction. A method for attenuation correction without a transmission scan has been developed and tested with the system [62].

Patients are imaged in the prone position, which is possible due to the existence of a breast aperture in the patient table. This allows to image regions close to the chest wall without breast compression.

The preliminary results using a 1 mm in diameter ^{22}Na point like source results of 1.6 mm FWHM axial and 1.9 transaxial in the center of the FoV and less than 3 mm FWHM in most other parts of the FoV (axial) [12, 63]. The system sensitivity at the FoV center and with a wide energy window of 250-759 keV is 1 %.

A pilot study was recently conducted with 32 invasive breast cancer patients to assess the feasibility of the system for tumor detection and characterization [64]. The system sensitivity for primary tumor visualization was 97%, which equals whole body PET-CT in the same study. This included lesions close to the chest wall.

4. Conclusions

With two commercially available PEM scanners, there is now data from several clinical studies that confirm the high sensitivity and specificity values for PEM in different clinical situations [65, 66]. These data also allow a direct comparison with other techniques such as PET and MRI and seem to indicate that the promise of molecular imaging with dedicated instruments as a valuable adjunct technique for mammography holds true.

Author details

Mónica Vieira Martins[1,2]

Address all correspondence to: mvmartins@estgp.pt

1 Polytechnic Institute of Portalegre, Portalegre, Portugal

2 Instituto de Biofísica e Engenharia Biomédica,Faculdade de Ciências, Universidade de Lisboa, Lisboa, Portugal

http://dx.doi.org/10.5772/60452

References

[1] Wahl RL. Current status of PET in breast cancer imaging, staging, and therapy. Semin Roentgenol. 2001 Jul;36(3):250–60.

[2] Gopalan D, Bomanji JB, Costa DC, Ell PJ. Nuclear Medicine in Primary Breast Cancer Imaging. Clin Radiol. 2002 Jul;57(7):565–74.

[3] Levin CS. Primer on molecular imaging technology. Eur J Nucl Med Mol Imaging. 2005 Dec;32 Suppl 2(14):S325–45.

[4] Bayley DL, Karp JS, Surti S. Physics and Instrumentation in PET. Positron Emission Tomography - Physics, Instrumentation and Scanners. Springer-Verlag; 2003.

[5] Defrise M, Kinahan PE, Christian M. Image Reconstruction Algorithms in PET. Positron Emission Tomography - Physics, Instrumentation and Scanners. Springer-Verlag; 2003.

[6] Korzhik M, Fedorov A, Annenkov A, Borissevitch A, Dossovitski A, Missevitch O, et al. Development of scintillation materials for PET scanners. Nucl Instruments Methods Phys Res Sect A Accel Spectrometers, Detect Assoc Equip. 2007 Feb;571(1-2):122–5.

[7] Humm JL, Rosenfeld A, Del Guerra A. From PET detectors to PET scanners. Eur J Nucl Med Mol Imaging. 2003 Nov;30(11):1574–97.

[8] Bruyndonckx P, Léonard S, Liu J, Tavernier S, Szupryczynski P, Fedorov A. Study of Spatial Resolution and Depth of Interaction of APD-Based PET Detector Modules Using Light Sharing Schemes. IEEE Trans Nucl Sci. 2003;50(5):1415–9.

[9] Thompson CJ, Cayouette F, Jolly D, Kecani S. A prototype modular detector design for high resolution positron emission mammography imaging. IEEE Trans Nucl Sci. 2003 Oct;50(5):1624–9.

[10] Pichler BJ, Ziegler SI. Photodetectors. In: Wernick M, Aarsvold JN, editors. Emission Tomography - the Fundamentals of PET and SPECT. Elsevier Academic Press; 2004.

[11] Macdonald L, Edwards J, Lewellen T, Haseley D, Rogers J, Kinahan P. Clinical Imaging Characteristics of the Positron Emission Mammography Camera: PEM Flex Solo II. J Nucl Med. 2009;50(10):1666–75.

[12] Moliner L, Gonzalez AJ, Soriano A, Sanchez F, Correcher C, Orero A, et al. Design and evaluation of the MAMMI dedicated breast PET. Med Phys Phys. 2012;39(9):5393–6404.

[13] Thompson CJ, Murthy K, Weinberg IN, Mako F. Feasibility study for Positron Emission Mammography. Med Phys. 1994;21(4):529–38.

[14] Thompson C., Murthy K, Picard Y, Weinberg IN, Mako F. Positron Emission Mammography (PEM) - a promising technique for detecting breast cancer. IEEE Trans Nucl Sci. 1995;42(4):1012–7.

[15] Bergman AM, Thompson C., Murthy K, Robar J., Clancy RL. Co-registration of positron emission mammography (pem) images and x-ray mammograms. IEEE Nuclear Science Symposium - Conference Record. 1997. p. 1812–6.

[16] Robar JL, Thompson CJ, Murthy IS, Clancy R, Bergman AM. Construction and calibration of detectors for high-resolution metabolic breast cancer imaging. Nucl Instruments Methods Phys Res - Sect A Accel Spectrometers Detect Assoc Equip. 1997;392(1-3):402–6.

[17] Robar J., Thompson CJ, Murthy K, Clancy RL, Bergman AM. Correction of spatial distortion, gain nonuniformity and efficiency variation in positron emission mammography. IEEE Nuclear Science Symposium - Conference Record. 1996. p. 1206–10.

[18] Murthy K, Aznar M, Thompson CJ, Loutfi A, Lisbona R, Gagnon JH. Results of Preliminary Clinical Trials of the Positron Emission Mammography System PEM-I: A Dedicated Breast Imaging System Producing Glucose Metabolic Images Using FDG. J Nucl Med. 1994;41(11):1851–8.

[19] Murthy K, Aznar M, Bergman AM, Thompson CJ, Robar JL, Lisbona R, et al. Positron Emission Mammographic Instrument: Initial Results. Radiology. 2000;215(1):280–5.

[20] Murthy K, Jolly D, Aznar M, Thompson CJ, Sciascia P, Loutfi A, et al. Quantification in positron emission mammography (PEM) with planar detectores: contrast resolution measurements using a custom breast phantom and novel spherical hot spots. IEEE Trans Nucl Sci. 1999;46(6):2192–6.

[21] Wollenweber SD, Williams RC, Beylin D, Dolinsky S, Weinberg IN. Investigation of the Quantitative Capabilities of a Positron Emission Mammography System. IEEE Nuclear Science Symposium - Conference Record. 2004. p. 8700–2.

[22] Weinberg IN, Stepanov PY, Beylin D, Anashkin E, Lauckner K, Yarnall S, et al. PEM-2400 – a Biopsy-Ready PEM Scanner with Real-Time X-Ray Correlation Capability. IEEE Nuclear Science Symposium - Conference Record. 2003. p. 1128–30.

[23] Weinberg I, David B, Steve Y, Anashkin E, Dolinsky S, Zavarzin V, et al. Applications of a PET Device with 1.5 mm FWHM Intrinsic Spatial Resolution to Breast Cancer Imaging. IEEE International Symposium on Biomedical Imaging: from Macro to Nano. 2004. p. 1396–9.

[24] Levine EA, Freimanis RI, Perrier ND, Morton K, Lesko NM, Bergman S, et al. Positron Emission Mammography: Initial Clinical Results. Ann Surg Oncol. 2003 Jan; 10(1):86–91.

[25] Tafra L, Cheng Z, Uddo J, Lobrano MB, Stein W, Berg W a, et al. Pilot clinical trial of 18F-fluorodeoxyglucose positron-emission mammography in the surgical management of breast cancer. Am J Surg. 2005 Oct;190(4):628–32.

[26] Raylman RR, Majewski S, Wojcik R, Weisenberger AG, Kross B, Popov V, et al. An Apparatus for Positron Emission Mammography Guided Biopsy. IEEE Nuclear Science Symposium - Conference Record. 1999. p. 1323–7.

[27] Raylman RR, Majewski S, Wojcik R, Weisenberger AG, Kross B, Popov V. Coincidences, Compton Scatter, and Object Size in Positron Emission Mammography (PEM) Imaging. IEEE Trans Nucl Sci. 2001;48(3):913–23.

[28] Raylman RR, Majewski S, Weisenberger AG, Popov V, Wojcik R, Kross B, et al. Positron Emission Mammography – Guided Breast Biopsy. J Nucl Med. 2001;42(6):960–6.

[29] Smith MF, Majewski S, Weisenberger AG, Kieper DA, Raylman RR, Turkington TG. Analysis of Factors Affecting Positron Emission Mammography (PEM) Image Formation. IEEE Nuclear Science Symposium - Conference Record. 2002. p. 2253–7.

[30] Smith MF, Raylman RR, Majewski S, Weisenberger AG. Positron emission mammography with tomographic acquisition using dual planar detectors: initial evaluations. Phys Med Biol. 2004;49(11):2437–52.

[31] Raylman RR, Virginia W, Smith MF, Kinahan PE, Majewski S. Quantification of radiotracer uptake with a dedicated breast PET imaging system. Med Phys. 2008;35(11): 4989–97.

[32] Raylman RR, Abraham J, Hazard H, Koren C, Filburn S, Schreiman JS, et al. Initial clinical test of a breast-PET scanner. J Med Imaging Radiat Oncol. 2011 Mar;55(1):58–64.

[33] Turkington TG, Majewski S, Weisenberger AG, Popov V, Smith MF, Sampson WH, et al. A Large Field of View Positron Emission Mammography Imager. IEEE Nuclear Science Symposium - Conference Record. 2003. p. 1883–6.

[34] Rosen EL, Turkington TG, Soo MS, Baker JA, Coleman RE. Radiology Detection of Primary Breast Carcinoma with a Dedicated, Large-Field-of-View FDG PET Mammography Device: Initial Experience. Radiology. 2005;234(2):527–34.

[35] Doshi NK, Shao Y, Silverman RW, Cherry SR. Design and evaluation of an LSO PET detector for breast cancer imaging. Med Phys. 2000;27(7):1535–43.

[36] Doshi NK, Silverman RW, Shao Y, Cherry SR. maxPET: A Dedicated Mammary and Axillary Region PET Imaging System for Breast Cancer. IEEE Trans Nucl Sci. 2001;48(3):811–5.

[37] Lamare F, Bowen SL, Visvikis D, Cortes P, Wu Y, Tran V, et al. Design Simulation of a Rotating Dual-Headed PET / CT Scanner for Breast Imaging. IEEE Nuclear Science Symposium - Conference Record. 2005. p. 1524–9.

[38] Wang G, Huber JS, Moses WW, Qi J, Member S, Choong W. Characterization of the LBNL PEM Camera. IEEE Trans Nucl Sci. 2006;53(3):1129–35.

[39] Qi J, Kuo C, Huesman RH, Klein GJ, Moses WW, Member S, et al. Comparison of Rectangular and Dual-Planar Positron Emission Mammography Scanners. IEEE Nuclear Science Symposium - Conference Record. 2002. p. 1246–50.

[40] Qi J, Klein GJ, Huesman RH, Member S. Image Properties of List-Mode Likelihood Reconstruction for a Rectangular Positron Emission Mammograph With DOI Measurements. IEEE Trans Nucl Sci. 2001;48(4):1343–9.

[41] Moses WW, Derenzo SE, Melcher CL, Manente RA. Room temperature LSO pin photodiode PET detector module that measures depth of interaction. IEEE Trans Nucl Sci. 1995;42(4):1085–9.

[42] Wang G, Member S, Huber JS, Moses WW, Member S, Choong W, et al. Calibration of a PEM Detector With Depth of Interaction Measurement. IEEE Trans Nucl Sci. 2004;51(3):775–81.

[43] Virador PRG, Moses WW, Huesman RH, Zatsiorsky VM. Reconstruction in PET Cameras with Irregular Sampling and Depth of Interaction Capability *. IEEE Trans Nucl Sci. 1998;45(3):1225–30.

[44] Virador PRG, Moses WW, Huesman RH, Zatsiorsky VM. 3D Reconstruction in PET Cameras with Irregular Sampling and Depth of Interaction. IEEE Trans Med Imaging. 2001;48(4):1524.

[45] Huesman RH, Klein GJ, Moses WW, Qi J, Reutter BW, Virador PRG. List-Mode Maximum-Likelihood Reconstruction Applied to Positron Emission Mammography (PEM) with Irregular Sampling. IEEE Trans Med Imaging. 2000;19(5):532–7.

[46] Qi J, Huesman RH. Lesion Detection and Quantitation of Positron Emission Mammography. IEEE Nuclear Science Symposium - Conference Record. 2002. p. 2248–52.

[47] Guerra A Del, Belcari N, Bencivelli W, Motta A, Righi S, Vaiano A, et al. Monte CArlo Study and Experimental Measurements of Breast Tumor Detectability with the YAP-PEMM prototype. IEEE Nuclear Science Symposium - Conference Record. 2003. p. 1887–91.

[48] Belcari N, Camarda M, Guerra A Del, Herbert D, Motta A, Vaiano A, et al. Development of a planar head PEM system based on an array of PSPMT and YAP crystals. IEEE Nuclear Science Symposium - Conference Record. 2004. p. 2179–82.

[49] Motta A, Guerra A del, Belcari N, Moehrs S, Panetta D, Righi S, et al. Fast 3D-EM reconstruction using Planograms for stationary planar positron emission mammography camera. Comput Med imaging Graph. 2005 Dec;29(8):587–96.

[50] Brasse D, Kinahan PE, Clackdoyle R, Defrise M, Comtat C, Townsend DW. List-Mode Maximum-Likelihood Reconstruction Applied to Positron Emission Mammography (PEM) with Irregular Sampling. IEEE Trans Med Imaging. 2004;23(4):413–25.

[51] Albuquerque E, Almeida FG, Auffray E, Barbosa J, Bastos AL, Bexiga V, et al. An overview of the Clear-PEM breast imaging scanner. 2008 IEEE Nuclear Science Symposium Conference Record. Ieee; 2008. p. 5616–8.

[52] Amaral P, Bruyndonckx P, Carriço B, Ferreira M, Luyten J, Moura R, et al. Long-term stability of the Clear-PEM detector modules. Nucl Instruments Methods Phys Res Sect A Accel Spectrometers, Detect Assoc Equip. 2007 Feb;571(1-2):488–92.

[53] Abreu MC, Aguiar JD, Almeida FG, Almeida P, Bento P, Carriço B, et al. Design and Evaluation of the Clear-PEM Scanner for Positron Emission Mammography. IEEE Trans Nucl Sci. 2006;53(1):71–7.

[54] Bento P, Gonçalves F, Leong C, Lousã P, Nobre J, Rego J, et al. Performance Simulation Studies of the Clear-PEM DAQ / Trigger System. IEEE Trans Nucl Sci. 2006;53(4):2102–11.

[55] Trindade A, Almeida P, Ferreira NC, Martins M V, Matela N, Oliveira N, et al. Breast Cancer Imaging Studies by Monte Carlo Simulation with Clear – PEM. IEEE Nuclear Science Symposium - Conference Record. 2005. p. 2103–7.

[56] Martins M V, Matela N, Oliveira N, Trindade A, Rodrigues P, Ferreira N, et al. Clear-PEM data reconstruction using STIR. Eur J Nucl Med Mol Imag. 2005;32(S1):S34.

[57] Cao L, Bugalho R, Matela N, Martins M V, Almeida P, Peter J, et al. List-Mode Maximum-Likelihood Reconstruction for the ClearPEM System. IEEE Nuclear Science Symposium - Conference Record. 2011. p. 4171–4.

[58] Abrantes M, Almeida P, Botelho F, Bugalho R, Carvalho S, Ferreira CS, et al. Clear-PEM scanners: performance results and studies in preclinical environment. IEEE Nuclear Science Symposium - Conference Record. 2011. p. 3291–5.

[59] Cucciati G, Auffray E, Bugalho R, Cao L, Vara N Di, Farina F, et al. Development of ClearPEM-Sonic, a multimodal mammography system for PET and Ultrasound. J Instrum. 2014 Mar 6;9(03):C03008–C03008.

[60] Frisch B, Dkfz P, Bugalho R, Neves J, Silva JC, Silva R. Development of ClearPEM-Sonic - a Multimodal Positron Emission Mammograph and Ultrasound Scanner. IEEE Nuclear Science Symposium - Conference Record. 2011. p. 2267–72.

[61] Fowler AM. A Molecular Approach to Breast Imaging. J Nucl Med. 2014;55(2):177–80.

[62] Soriano A, González A, Orero A, Moliner L, Carles M, Sánchez F, et al. Attenuation correction without transmission scan for the MAMMI breast PET. Nucl Instruments

Methods Phys Res Sect A Accel Spectrometers, Detect Assoc Equip. 2011 Aug; 648:S75–S78.

[63] Moliner L, Benlloch JM, Carles M, Correcher C, González AJ, Orero A, et al. Performance Characteristics of the MAMMI PEMT Scanner Based on NEMA NU 2-2007. 2010 IEEE Nuclear Science Symposium Conference Record (NSS/MIC), . 2010. p. 2591–4.

[64] Koolen BB, Aukema TS, González AJ, Vogel W V., Caballero L, Peeters MJTFDV, et al. First clinical experience with a dedicated PET for hanging breast molecular imaging. Q J Nucl Med Mol Imaging. 2013;57(1):92–100.

[65] Berg WA, Madsen KS, Schilling K, Pisano ED, Larsen LH, Ozonoff A, et al. Breast Cancer: Comparative Effectiveness of Positron Emission Mammography and MR Imaging in Presurgical Planning. Radiology. 2011;258(1):59.

[66] Schilling K, Narayanan D, Kalinyak JE, The J, Velasquez MV, Kahn S, et al. Positron emission mammography in breast cancer presurgical planning: comparisons with magnetic resonance imaging. Eur J Nucl Med Mol Imaging. 2011 Jan;38(1):23–36.

Chapter 4

Digital Mammogram Enhancement

Michal Haindl and Václav Remeš

Additional information is available at the end of the chapter

http://dx.doi.org/10.5772/60988

1. Introduction

Three fully automatic methods for X-ray digital mammogram enhancement based on a fast analytical textural model are presented. These efficient single and double view enhancement methods are based on the underlying two-dimensional adaptive causal autoregressive texture model. The methods locally predict breast tissue texture from single or double view mammograms and enhance breast tissue abnormalities, such as the sign of a developing cancer, using the estimated model prediction statistics. The double-view mammogram enhancement is based on the cross-prediction of two mutually registered left and right breasts' mammograms or alternatively a temporal sequence of mammograms. The single-view mammogram enhancement is based on modeling prediction error in case of not the both breasts' mammograms being available.

Breast cancer is the most common type of cancer among middle-aged women in most developed countries [1, 2]. Almost one woman in ten grows a breast cancer in her life. According to the American Cancer Society [3] about 232 670 new cases of invasive breast cancer will be diagnosed in women and about 40 000 women will die from breast cancer in US alone. US mortality rate is 30% and European mortality rate is 45% [4].

To lower the mortality rate, women in the developed countries usually regularly attend a preventive mammography screening. However, around 25% of radiologically visible cancers are missed by the radiologists at screening [5]. This means that millions of cancer cases are missed and therefore even a slightest improvement in the detection methods could have a huge impact and save many lives.

The biggest problem with current Computer-Aided Diagnosis (CAD) systems is their large false negative rate and an even larger false positive rate. Most CAD systems (e.g., [1, 6]) point out 2-3 regions of interest (ROIs) per mammogram on average. Taking into account that there are about 8 malignant mammograms in 1000 [5], the radiologists consider the current CAD systems as misleading.

An alternative way is to automatically enhance mammograms to support radiologists with their visual mammogram evaluation. Several mammogram enhancement methods have been published [7–14]. Salvado and Roque [10] use wavelet analysis to detect microcalcifications, Dippel et al. [8] compare the merits of using either Laplacian pyramids or wavelet analysis for whole mammogram enhancement, Sakellaropoulos et al. [9] designed an adaptive wavelet based method for enhancing the contrast of the whole mammograms. Mencattini et al. [13] selectively enhance segmented mammograms regions using wavelet transformation.

An approach to diagnostic evaluation of screening mammograms based on local statistical Gaussian mixture textural models was proposed in [14]. The local evaluation tool has the form of a multivariate probability density of gray levels in a suitably chosen search window. First, the density function in the form of a Gaussian mixture is estimated from data obtained by scanning the mammogram with the search window. The estimated mixture is evaluated at each position and displays the corresponding log-likelihood value as a gray level at the window center. The resulting log-likelihood image closely correlates with the structural details of the original mammogram and emphasizes unusual places, but the method is very computationally demanding.

Radiologists regularly compare the bilateral mammogram pairs during mammogram screening in search for breast abnormalities. The mutual mammograms enhancement requires accurate registration of both breast X-ray images, which is difficult due to their elasticity. Marias et al. [15, 16] use thin-plate spline transformation [17] to align the breasts and then use wavelet based feature detection to find internal landmarks. Thin-plate spline based approach is also used by Wirth et al. in [18]. Hachama [19] deals only with the comparison of temporal mammograms based on a general method for registering images with the presence of abnormalities. However, it needs the prior abnormalities distribution knowledge. The registration and transformation are based on the Bayesian maximum a posteriori probability approach and minimization of the registration and deformation energy.

The novelty of our presented method is that whereas other alternative methods usually use simple pixel difference or trivial statistics like cross-correlation to compare the left and right images, we use the mammograms of one breast as a learning sample for the 2DCAR breast texture model [20, 21] and then try to analyze the other mammogram based on this acquired information. Using the 2DCAR model for bilateral comparison, we achieve a result which is robust to inaccurate registration, very fast, and which gives improved enhancement results compare to just a single-view analysis even using similar local texture modeling.

2. Public mammogram databases

There are not many publicly available mammogram databases [22–26], older databases like DDSM, MIAS are digitized from the X-ray films, while newer databases like INbreast are already digitaly acquired.

The Digital Database for Screening Mammography (DDSM) [24] http://marathon.csee.usf.edu/Mammography/Database.html is a database of digitized from original X-ray filmscreen in different resolutions and with associated ground truth and other information. This database was completed in 1999 and contains mammograms from four different sources using four different digitizers (DBA M2100 ImageClear, Howtek 960, Lumisys 200 Laser, Howtek MultiRad850) and 12 or 16 bits quantization. The database contains normal, benign, and histologically proven cancerous mammograms in four different views (left and right cranio-caudal (CC) and medio-lateral oblique (MLO)). It contains breast imaging reporting and data system (BI-RADS) keywords and the American College of Radiology (ACR) tissue codes (Table 1).

ACR	Tissue density description	BI-RADS	Tumor description
-	unspecified	BI-RADS 0	unspecified
ACR-1	fat transparent system	BI-RADS 1	normal
ACR-2	fibroid glands system	BI-RADS 2	benign
ACR-3	heterogeneously dense	BI-RADS 3	probably benign
ACR-3/4	dense	BI-RADS 4	suspiciously abnormal
ACR-4	extremely dense	BI-RADS 5	malignant

Table 1. ACR and BI-RADS codes.

The Mammographic Image Analysis Society Digital Mammogram Database (miniMIAS) [22] is also digitized to 50 microns per pixel from the original X-ray filmscreen mammograms by the scanning microdensitometer SCANDIG3. MIAS mammographic images are available via the Pilot European Image Processing Archive (PEIPA) at the University of Essex http://peipa.essex.ac.uk/ipa/info/mias.html.

The LLNL/UCSF database ftp://gdo-biomed.ucllnl.org/pub/mammo-db/ [23] contains 198 digitized films from 50 patients with 4 views per patient (but only 2 views from one mastectomy case).

The INbreast database [26] is a mammographic database, with images acquired at a Breast Centre, located in a University Hospital (Hospital de São João, Breast Centre, Porto, Portugal). INbreast has a total of 115 cases (410 images) of which 90 cases are from women with both breasts (4 images per case) and 25 cases are from mastectomy patients (2 images per case). Several types of lesions (masses, calcifications, asymmetries, and distortions) are included. Accurate contours made by specialists are also provided in the XML format.

The recent BancoWeb LAPIMO Database http://lapimo.sel.eesc.usp.br/bancoweb/ [27] was acquired in two hospitals using Senographe 500t and Senographe 600t mammographs and digitized by using two laser scanners Lumiscan 50 and Lumiscan 75.

The overview of major features of the public mammographic databases are listed in the following Table 2.

3. Mammogram enhancement methods

The mammogram enhancement methods can be roughly categorized into frequency based and spatial based methods. The frequency based methods [7, 9, 28, 29] use mostly some wavelet multiscale decomposition with modified wavelet coefficients to enhance mammogram contrast. The spatial methods [14, 30] use some nonlinear or adaptive linear filters.

We have implemented four representative mammogram enhancement methods from several published alternatives [7–10, 10–14] to compare with our novel adaptive probabilistic mammogram enhancement method.

	DDSM ([24])	INbreast ([26])	miniMIAS ([22])	LLNL ([23])	LAPIMO ([27])
n_{mam}	10480	410	322	198	1473
n_{views}	4	4	2	4	4
n_{gl}	16/12	14	8	12	12
x *resolution*	1411 – 5641	2560 – 3328	1024		
y *resolution*	3256 – 7111	3328 – 4084	1024		
normal	695	70	204	38	294
↓ *benign*	141	116		128	994
benign	870	44	66		
malignant	914	180	52	32	112
density	*ACR*	*ACR*	*own scale*	*no*	*no*
BI-RADS	*yes*	*yes*	*no*	*no*	*yes*

Table 2. Public Mammogram Databases: where (n_{mam}) is the number of mammograms, (n_{views}) number of views, (n_{gl}) number of gray levels in bits, and ↓is benign without callback.

3.1. Histogram equalization

The well known gray scale image enhancement technique is histogram equalization [31], which is based on the idea of forcing the enhanced image histogram to be uniform. This is a popular technique for contrast enhancement because because of its simplicity and effectivity. However, it may overenhance the noises and sharp regions in the original images.

3.2. Matting-based enhancement

The enhancement method based on the idea of image matting was published in [32]. It works based on the idea that mammographic images (Y) are a superposition of some background adipose tissue (B) and the interesting part, which would be the mammary glands and other breast structures (G).

$$Y = Gc + B(1 - c) \quad (1)$$

The enhancement method then selectively subtracts the background tissues from the superposition, thus creating the enhanced image.

To enable this, the authors had to estimate the background (B) and the opacity alpha value for each pixel by which it is blended with the rest of the image (c). In this method the background is set as a constant value for the whole image represented by the 85% percentile of grey values of the breast part of the image.

3.3. Nonlinear unsharp masking

A nonlinear unsharp masking (NLUM) combined with nonlinear filtering for mammogram enhancement was introduced in [33]. The method embeds different types of filters into the nonlinear filtering operator within the 3×3 window which fuses the enhanced and original mammogram data. The unsharp masking emphasizes high-frequencies of the signal either by subtracting a low-pass filtered signal from its original or adding a scaled high-frequency factor to the measured original. NLUM eight parameters are optimized using the proposed second-derivative-like measure of enhancement (SDME) [33].

http://dx.doi.org/10.5772/60988

3.4. Direct contrast enhancement

An enhancement method based on wavelet transformation was described in [29]. The method performs a multi-level 2D wavelet transfomation and at each level the 3 highpass components are divided by the lowpass-lowpass component, getting a directional contrast estimate, which is further multiplied by a constant contrast enhancement factor λ. Starting at the deepest level of the transform, the inverse transform is performed one scale at a time. For each scale level, before the inverse transform step, the 3 modified components are multiplied by the newly computed lowpass component. This way the authors achieve a contrast enhancement without the introduction of too much of additional noise.

4. Probabilistic mammogram enhancement

These our methods use Markovian texture models for the analysis of local texture characteristics and enhancing breast tissue abnormalities such as microcalcifications and masses which could be the sign of a developing cancer. We make the presumption that left and right breasts are architecturally symmetrical. This presumption is indeed reasonable, since radiologists frequently compare double-view mammograms to find asymmetrical parts, which could indicate a developing cancer. The texture based symmetry detection neither needs to assume the pixel-wise correspondence of the both breast images, nor their ideal sub-pixel registration inside the breast area.

The double-view methods consist of three major steps: registration, model parameters adaptive estimation, and the cross-prediction based analysis.

4.1. Mammogram registration

The registration process is described for mammographic MLO views, but it can be easily adapted also for CC views. Since we compare the images based on textural features rather than pixel-wise, we do not require as precise registration as other methods, and can use a simple registration based on the affine transformation.

Three reference points are needed for the affine transformation (Figure 1). We chose the nipple and one point above and one below that are closest to the pectoral muscle.

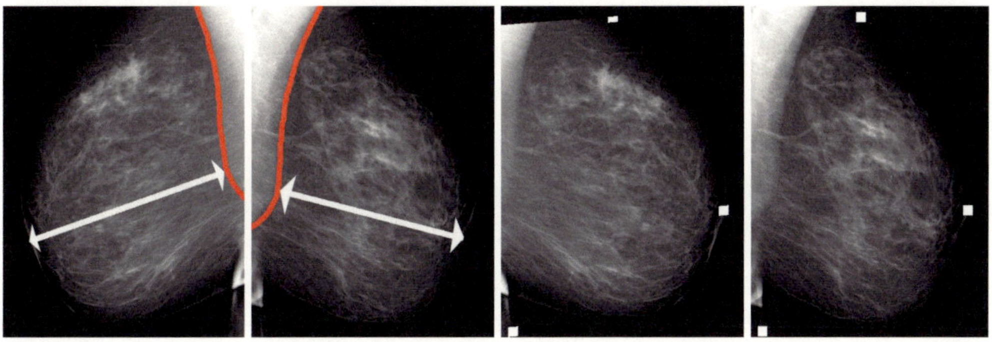

Figure 1. Registered mammograms with visible reference points.

The nipple is located using the heuristic method described in [34]. It works on the idea of the nipple being a point on the skin-line of the breast which is the most distant from the line of the pectoral muscle. After the candidates for the nipple reference points have been found in both the mammograms, the position of the reference point can still slightly differ in both images. Therefore, we adjust their position by searching the neighborhood on the skin line of the breast for the most correlated window.

The remaining reference point candidates have to be further adjusted as well. Since the bilateral mammograms usually do not cover the same area of the breast, some anatomical parts of the breast can be seen only in one of the images and therefore the reference points wouldn't match. To make up for this problem, we measure the distance of the points to the nipple, weighted by the nipples distance to the pectoral muscle. The weighting compensates for the differences of positioning of the breast in the mammogram which could result in one image displaying the breast bigger than the other. We then adjust the corresponding reference points, so that they are on the skin line with the most similar weighted distance to the nipple possible.

Having found the reference points, the affine transformation is performed. Figure 1 in the leftmost images shows the images of right and left breast with marked line of the pectoral muscle (colored in red) and the distance from the pectoral muscle to the nipple. The rightmost images show the registered breasts with the reference points painted as white squares with the right breast (shown on the left side) transformed to match the left breast.

4.2. Adaptive textural model

The X-ray mammographic tissue is locally modeled by its dedicated independent Gaussian noise-driven autoregressive random field two-dimensional texture model (2DCAR), which is a rare exception among Markovian random field model family that can be completely analytically solved [35, 36]. Apart from that, this descriptive model has good modeling performance, all statistics can be evaluated recursively, and the model is very fast to evaluate.

The 2DCAR random field is a Markovian family of random variables with a joint probability density on the set of all possible realizations Y of the $M \times N$ lattice I, subject to the following condition:

$$p(Y \mid \gamma, \sigma^{-2}) = (2\pi\sigma^2)^{-\frac{(MN-1)}{2}} \exp\left\{\frac{-1}{2} tr \left\{\sigma^{-2} \begin{pmatrix} -\alpha \\ \gamma^T \end{pmatrix}^T \tilde{V}_{MN-1} \begin{pmatrix} -\alpha \\ \gamma^T \end{pmatrix}\right\}\right\} , \tag{2}$$

where α is a unit vector, $tr()$ is a trace of the corresponding matrix, and the following notation is used

$$\tilde{V}_{r-1} = \sum_{k=1}^{r-1} \begin{pmatrix} Y_k Y_k^T & Y_k X_k^T \\ X_k Y_k^T & X_k X_k^T \end{pmatrix} = \begin{pmatrix} \tilde{V}_{y(r-1)} & \tilde{V}_{xy(r-1)}^T \\ \tilde{V}_{xy(r-1)} & \tilde{V}_{x(r-1)} \end{pmatrix} .$$

Here, $r = [r_1, r_2, \phi]$ is spatial multiindex denoting history of movements on the rectangular lattice I, where r_1, r_2 are row and column indices, and the direction of the model development is $\phi \in \{0°, 45°, 90°, 135°, 180°, 225°, 270°, 315°\}$. The 2DCAR model can be expressed as a stationary causal uncorrelated noise-driven 2D autoregressive process:

$$Y_r = \gamma_\phi X_r + e_r \ , \tag{3}$$

where $\gamma_\phi = [a_1, \ldots, a_\eta]$ is the parameter vector, $\eta = cardinality(I_r^c)$, I_r^c denotes a causal (or alternatively unilateral) contextual neighborhood (i.e., all support pixels were previously visited and thus they are known). Elements in I_r^c do not need to be topological neighbours of each other, i.e., if s is a neighbour of r then $\exists t, t \in I$ located between r and s at a distance $\delta(r,t) < \delta(r,s)$ such as $t \notin I_r^c$. This type of a neighbourhood system is also called a functional neighbourhood system and its application is illustrated in Figure 2. Its optimal configuration can be found analytically using the Bayesian statistics see [36] for details. Furthermore, e_r denotes white Gaussian noise with zero mean and a constant but unknown variance σ^2, and X_r is a support vector of Y_{r-s} where $s \in I_r^c$. The method uses a locally adaptive version of this 2DCAR model [36], where its recursive statistics are modified by an exponential forgetting factor, i.e., a constant smaller than 1 which is used to weight the older data.

4.2.1. Parameter estimation

Parameter estimation of the 2DCAR model using either the maximum likelihood, the least square or Bayesian methods can be found analytically. The Bayesian parameter estimates of the 2DCAR model using the normal-gamma parameter prior are:

$$\hat{\gamma}_{r-1}^T = V_{x(r-1)}^{-1} V_{xy(r-1)} \ , \tag{4}$$

$$\hat{\sigma}_{r-1}^2 = \frac{\lambda_{(r-1)}}{\beta(r)} \ , \tag{5}$$

where

$$\lambda_{(r-1)} = V_{y(r-1)} - V_{xy(r-1)}^T V_{x(r-1)}^{-1} V_{xy(r-1)} \ ,$$
$$V_{(r-1)} = \tilde{V}_{(r-1)} + V_{(0)} \ ,$$
$$\beta(r) = \beta(0) + r - 1 \ ,$$

and $\beta(0)$ is an initialization constant and submatrices in $V_{(0)}$ are from the parameter prior. The parameter estimates (4),(5) can also be evaluated recursively [36] using the proces history $(Y^{(r-1)})$. The posterior probability density [36] of the model is:

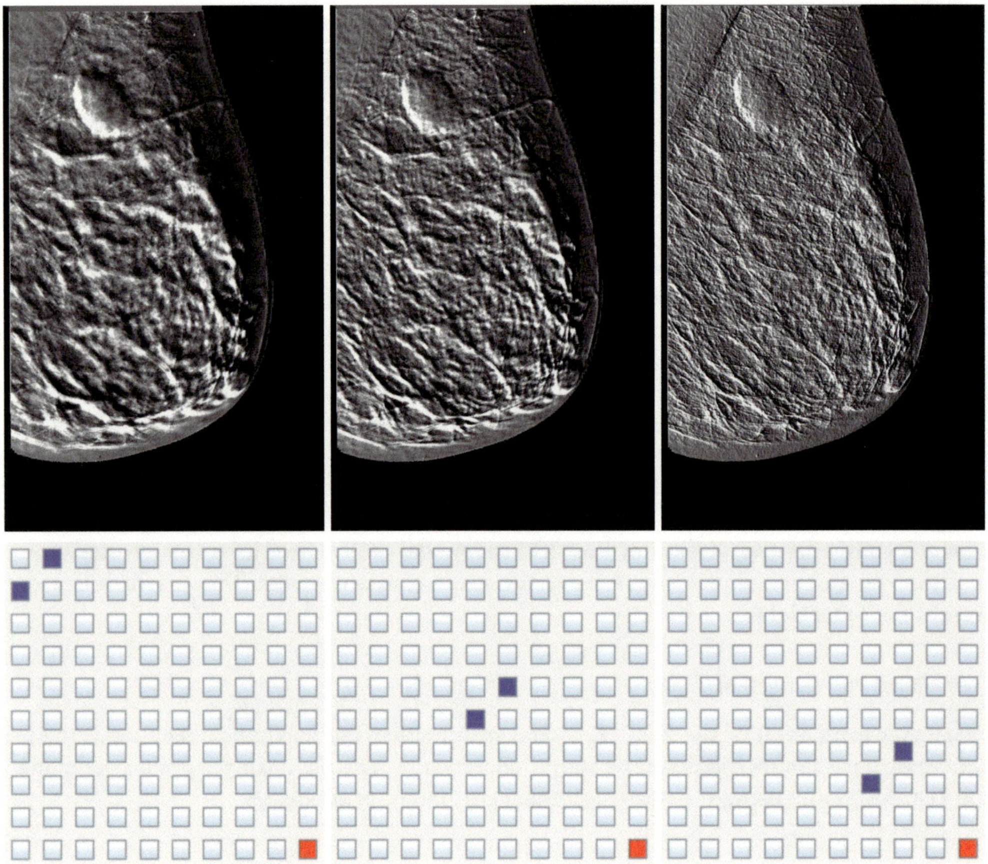

Figure 2. Single-view MLO mammogram enhancement using different functional neighbourhoods consecutively rightwards - 9, 5, and 3 pixel neighbourhood distance from the enhanced pixel (blue pixels - bottom row).

$$p(Y_r \mid Y^{(r-1)}, \hat{\gamma}_{r-1}) = \frac{\Gamma(\frac{\beta(r)-\eta+3}{2})}{\Gamma(\frac{\beta(r)-\eta+2}{2})\ \pi^{\frac{1}{2}}\ (1 + X_r^T V_{x(r-1)}^{-1} X_r)^{\frac{1}{2}}\ |\lambda_{(r-1)}|^{\frac{1}{2}}} \left(1 + \frac{(Y_r - \hat{\gamma}_{r-1}X_r)^T \lambda_{(r-1)}^{-1} (Y_r - \hat{\gamma}_{r-1}X_r)}{1 + X_r^T V_{x(r-1)}^{-1} X_r}\right)^{-\frac{\beta(r)-\eta+3}{2}} \quad (6)$$

And the conditional mean value predictor of the one-step-ahead predictive posterior density (6) for the normal-gamma parameter prior is

$$E\left\{Y_r \mid Y^{(r-1)}\right\} = \hat{\gamma}_{r-1} X_r \ . \quad (7)$$

http://dx.doi.org/10.5772/60988

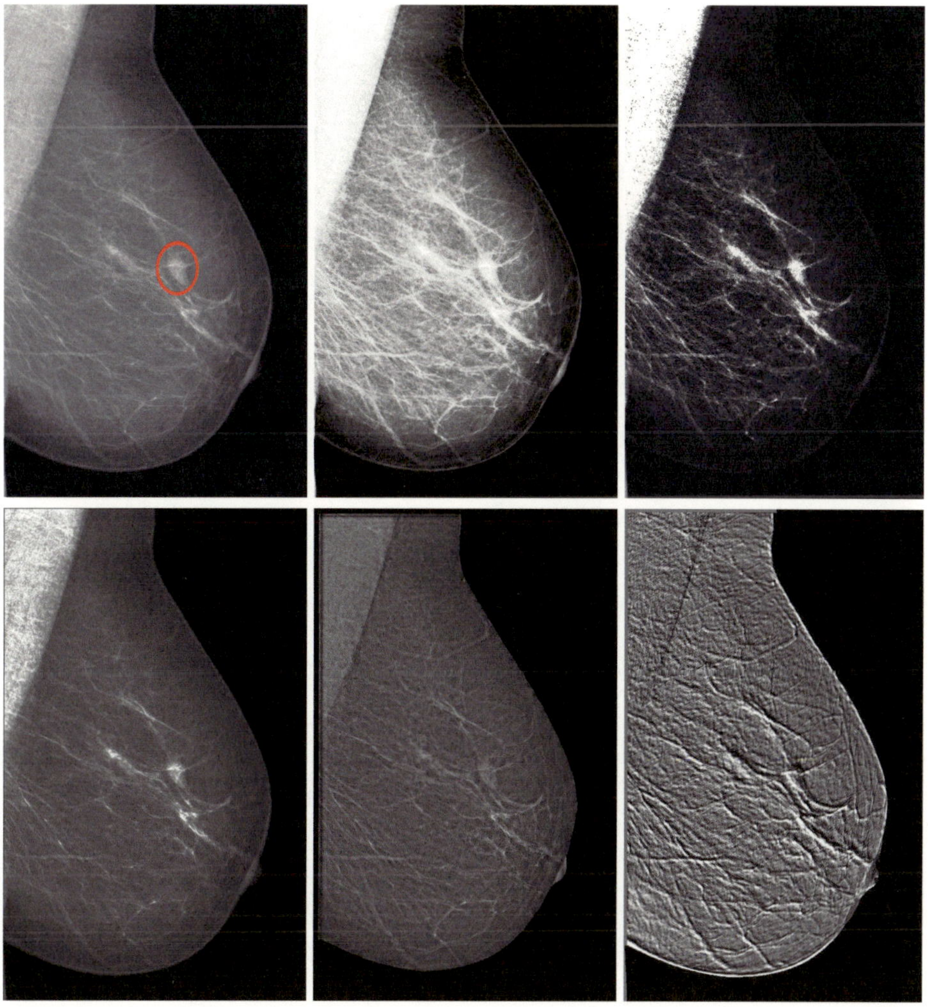

Figure 3. INbreast MLO mammogram enhancement comparison rightwards: the original mammogram, histogram equalization, [32], [33], [29], and the presented enhancement methods, respectively.

4.2.2. Prediction

The conditional mean value of the one-step-ahead predictive posterior density for the normal-gamma parameter prior is

$$E\left\{Y_r \mid Y^{(r-1)}\right\} = \hat{\gamma}_{r-1} X_r \ . \tag{8}$$

The predictor (8) is used only for single-view mammogram enhancement. For double-view mammograms where there are available both left and right breasts mammograms the method uses the cross-prediction (10),(11).

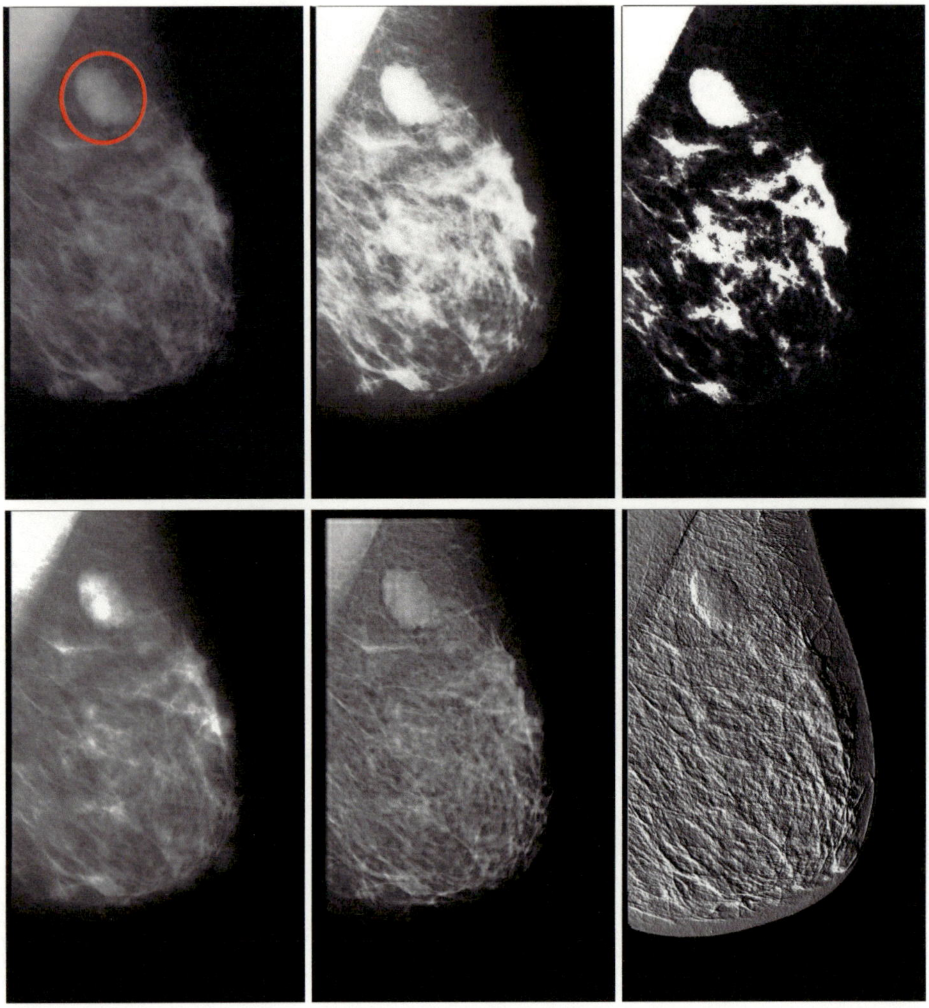

Figure 4. MIAS MLO mammogram enhancement comparison rightwards: the original mammogram, histogram equalization, [32], [33], [29], and the presented enhancement methods, respectively.

4.3. Enhancement methods

Let us denote two mutually registered (e.g., left and right breasts') mammograms Y and $\tilde{Y}$, the local 2DCAR model parameters estimates (4), (5) computed on the mammogram image Y $\hat{\gamma}^T_{r-1}, \hat{\sigma}^2_{r-1}$. The same parameter estimates (4), (5) computed on the other mammogram $\tilde{Y}$ are denoted $\tilde{\gamma}^T_{r-1}, \tilde{\sigma}^2_{r-1}$, and the corresponding support vector is $\tilde{X}_r$. The directional models are computed in the following angles $\phi \in \Phi = \{0°, 45°, 90°, 135°, 180°, 225°, 270°, 315°\}$.

4.3.1. Single-view enhancement

The single-view enhacement method is computed from up to eight directional models, i.e.,

http://dx.doi.org/10.5772/60988

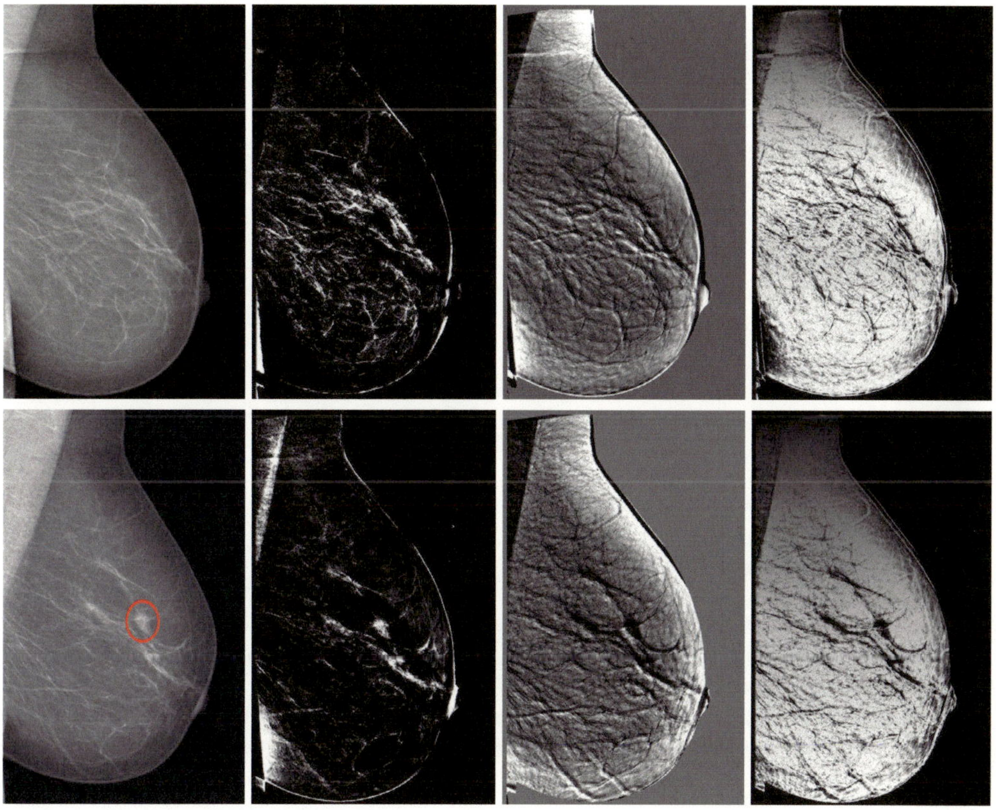

Figure 5. INbreast multiple-view MLO mammogram enhancement consecutively rightwards - ground truth, pixel difference between registered LMLO and RMLO, cross-predicted gradient, and cross-prediction probability density. The upper row contains LMLO, bottom row RMLO.

$$Y_r^{enh} = \sum_{\forall \phi \in \bar{\Phi}} (Y_{r+1} - \hat{\gamma}_{r-1} X_r) \ , \qquad (9)$$

where $\bar{\Phi} \subseteq \Phi$. All the enhanced values are normalized into the $0 - 255$ range.

4.3.2. Double-view enhancement

The double-view enhancement is based on statistics computed on one breast image and applied to the complementary one. The cross-prediction between images $Y, \tilde{Y}$ is computed as follows:

$$E\left\{ \tilde{Y}_r \,|\, Y^{(r-1)} \right\} = \hat{\gamma}_{r-1} \tilde{X}_r \qquad (10)$$

and the opposite direction cross-prediction is analogously

$$E\left\{Y_r \,|\, \tilde{Y}^{(r-1)}\right\} = \tilde{\gamma}_{r-1} X_r \ . \tag{11}$$

The enhanced mammograms are then the corresponding cross-prediction statistics images. The corresponding cross-prediction probability densities are $p(\tilde{Y}_r \,|\, \tilde{Y}^{(r-1)}, \hat{\gamma}_{r-1})$ and $p(Y_r \,|\, Y^{(r-1)}, \tilde{\gamma}_{r-1})$.

The proposed double-view enhancement methods are

$$Y_r^{com_1} = \sum_{\forall \phi \in \bar{\Phi}} \left(\tilde{Y}_{r+1} - \hat{\gamma}_{r-1} X_r\right) \ , \tag{12}$$

$$Y_r^{com_2} = \sum_{\forall \phi \in \bar{\Phi}} p(\tilde{Y}_r \,|\, \tilde{Y}^{(r-1)}, \hat{\gamma}_{r-1}) \ . \tag{13}$$

5. Experimental results

The comparative experimental results (Figures 3, 4) were tested on the miniMIAS database [22] and on the state-of-the-art public digital mammogram INbreast database [26]. Comparing the alternative methods (Section 3) with our proposed adaptive enhancement, it is clearly visible that whereas these methods enhance prevailingly contrast, our method enhances textural abnormalities in the breast tissue which is more useful for the radiologists.

Our adaptive enhancement methods were also successfully tested on the Digital Database for Screening Mammography (DDSM) from the University of South Florida [24]. These results are reported elsewhere.

The spatial textural model allows seamless and natural generalization into multiple-view mammogram enhancement (be it bilateral, as presented in Figures 5, 6, or temporal). Double-view medio-lateral oblique digital mammograms' enhancements from the INbreast database (Figure 5) and the miniMIAS database (Figure 6) show the cross-prediction based enhancement performance. Comparing the cross-prediction enhancements on Figures 5, 6 respectively with the same breast single-view enhancements on Figures 3, 4, the benefits of the cross-prediction are clearly visible.

Both our double-view enhancement methods are compared with the registered image pixel difference which is standardly used for comparison ([15, 18, 19])

$$\Delta Y_r = max\{Y_r^R - Y_r^L, 0\} \ . \tag{14}$$

This standard double-view enhancement method (Figures 5, 6 - second columns) is inferior compared to the both proposed double-view enhancement methods ((12), (13)) which simultaneously exhibit more contrast and increased details' visibility.

Finally, all three proposed enhancement methods are very fast - they can be computed on the presented mammograms with a standard PC in a matter of several seconds.

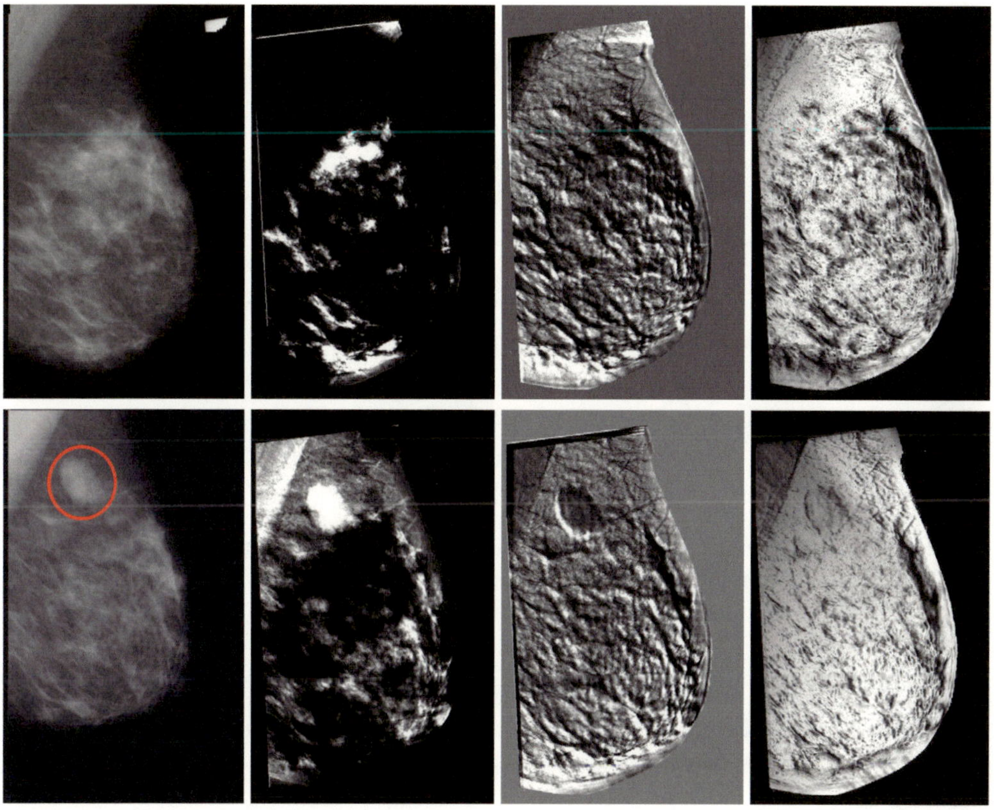

Figure 6. Multiple-view medio-lateral mammogram (INbreast) enhancement consecutively rightwards - ground truth, pixel difference between registered LMLO and RMLO, cross-predicted gradient, and cross-prediction probability density. The upper row contains LMLO, bottom row RMLO.

6. Conclusions

We proposed three novel fast methods for completely automatic mammogram enhancement which highlight regions of interest, detected as textural abnormalities. Cancerous areas typically manifest themselves in X-ray mammography as such textural defects which is advantageous for our methods in comparison with most alternative mammogram enhancement methods that primarily enhance only the image contrast. Thus the enhanced mammograms can help radiologists to decrease their false negative evaluation rate.

These methods are based on the underlying two-dimensional adaptive CAR texture model. Although the algorithms use random field type model, the model is very fast due to the efficient recursive model predictor estimation and therefore is much faster than the usual alternative Markov chain Monte Carlo estimation approach. The enhancement can be either single or double view depending on the available data. The single-view methods allow significant mammogram enhancement without the need of paired mammogram registration. The double-view methods benefit from mutual textural information in the registered bilateral breast pairs. Contrary to the simple pixel difference values or cross-correlations, the textural feature comparison brings increased robustness to registration inaccuracies inevitably encountered due to the elasticity of the breast. The double-view methods could alternatively be used for the enhancement of a temporal sequence of mammograms.

Acknowledgements

This research was supported by the Czech Science Foundation project GAČR 14-10911S.

Author details

Michal Haindl and Václav Remeš

The Institute of Information Theory and Automation of the Czech Academy of Sciences, Prague, Czech Republic

References

[1] Tweed, T.; Miguet, S. Automatic Detection of Regions of Interest in Mammographies Based on a Combined Analysis of Texture and Histogram. In *Pattern Recognition, 2002. Proceedings. 16th International Conference on*, Vol. 2; IEEE Computer Society: Los Alamitos, CA, USA, 2002.

[2] Qi, H.; Diakides, N. A. Thermal Infrared Imaging in Early Breast Cancer Detection - A Survey of Recent Research. In *Proceedings of the 25th Annual International Conference of the IEEE Engineering in Medicine and Biology Society*, Vol. 2; 2003.

[3] ACS, "Breast cancer facts & figures 2011 -? 2012", Technical Report, American cancer society, 2012.

[4] Kopans, D. B. *Radiology* 2010, *256*, 15–20.

[5] Taylor, P. and Champness, J. and Given-Wilson, R. and Johnston, K. and Potts, H., *Health Technology Assessment* 2005, *9*,.

[6] Haindl, M.; Mikeš, S.; Scarpa, G. Unsupervised Detection of Mammogram Regions of Interest. In *Knowledge-Based Intelligent Information and Engineering Systems*, Vol. 4694; Apolloni, B.; Howlett, R. J.; Jain, L., Eds.; Springer: 2007.

[7] Chang, C.-M.; Laine, A. *IEEE Transactions on Information Technology in Biomedicine* 1999, *3*, 32–46.

[8] Dippel, S.; Stahl, M.; Wiemker, R.; Blaffert, T. *Medical Imaging, IEEE Transactions on* 2002, *21*, 343–353.

[9] Sakellaropoulos, P.; Costaridou, L.; Panayiotakis, G. *Physics in medicine and biology* 2003, *48*, 787.

[10] Salvado, J.; Roque, B. Detection of calcifications in digital mammograms using wavelet analysis and contrast enhancement. In *Intelligent Signal Processing, 2005 IEEE International Workshop on*; 2005.

[11] Yan, Z.; Zhang, Y.; Liu, B.; Zheng, J.; Lu, L.; Xie, Y.; Liang, Z.; Li, J. Extracting hidden visual information from mammography images using conjugate image enhancement software. In *Information Acquisition, 2005 IEEE International Conference on*; IEEE: 2005.

[12] Thangavel, K.; Karnan, M.; Sivakumar, R.; Mohideen, A. *Graphics, Vision and Image Processing* 2007, 55–60.

[13] Mencattini, A.; Salmeri, M.; Lojacono, R.; Frigerio, M.; Caselli, F. *Instrumentation and Measurement, IEEE Transactions on* 2008, *57,* 1422–1430.

[14] Grim, J.; Somol, P.; Haindl, M.; Daneš, J. *IEEE Transactions on Image Processing* 2009, *18,* 765 - 773.

[15] Marias, K.; Behrenbruch, C. P.; Brady, M.; Parbhoo, S.; Seifalian, A. Multi-scale landmark selection for improved registration of temporal mammograms. In *International Workshop on Database Machines*; 2000.

[16] Marias, K. and Behrenbruch, C. and Parbhoo, S. and Seifalian, A. and Brady, M., *Medical Imaging, IEEE Transactions on* 2005, *24,* 782–790.

[17] Harder, R L and Desmarais, R N, *Journal of Aircraft* 1972, *9,* 189–191.

[18] Wirth, M. A.; Narhan, J.; Gray, D. A model for nonrigid mammogram registration using mutual information. In *In International Workshop on Digital Mammography*; 2002.

[19] Hachama, M. and Richard, F. and Desolneux, A., A mammogram registration technique dealing with outliers. In *Biomedical Imaging: Nano to Macro, 2006. 3rd IEEE International Symposium on*; 2006.

[20] Haindl, M.; Havlíček, V. A multiscale colour texture model. In *Pattern Recognition, 2002. Proceedings. 16th International Conference on*, Vol. 1; 2002.

[21] Haindl, M.; Šimberová, S. *Theory & Applications of Image Analysis* 1992, 306–315.

[22] Suckling, J. *et al.* The mammographic image analysis society digital mammogram database. In *2nd International Workshop on Digital Mammography*; International Congress Series Excerta Medica: 1994.

[23] LLNL, "Lawrence Livermore National Library / UCSF Digital Mammogram Database", Technical Report, Center for Health Care Technologies Livermore, Lawrence Livermore National Library, Livermore, CA, USA, 1995.

[24] Heath, M.; Bowyer, K.; Kopans, D.; Moore, R.; Kegelmeyer, P. The Digital Database for Screening Mammography. In *Proc. of the 5th Int. Workshop on Digital Mammography*; Medical Physics Publishing: 2000.

[25] Oliveira, J. E.; Gueld, M. O.; Araújo, A. d. A.; Ott, B.; Deserno, T. M. Toward a standard reference database for computer-aided mammography. In *Medical Imaging*; 2008.

[26] Moreira, I. C.; Amaral, I.; Domingues, I.; Cardoso, A.; Cardoso, M. J.; Cardoso, J. S. *Academic radiology* 2012, *19,* 236–248.

[27] Matheus, B. R. N.; Schiabel, H. *Journal of digital imaging* 2011, *24*, 500–506.

[28] Mencattini, A.; Caselli, F.; Salmeri, M.; Lojacono, R. Wavelet based adaptive algorithm for mammographic images enhancement and denoising. In *Image Processing, 2005. ICIP 2005. IEEE International Conference on*, Vol. 1; 2005.

[29] Tang, J.; Liu, X.; Sun, Q. *Selected Topics in Signal Processing, IEEE Journal of* 2009, *3*, 74–80.

[30] Dhawan, A. P.; Buelloni, G.; Gordon, R. *Medical Imaging, IEEE Transactions on* 1986, *5*, 8–15.

[31] Pratt, W. K. *Digital image processing: PIKS inside;* John Wiley & Sons, Inc: 2007.

[32] Wang, H.; Li, J.-B.; Wu, L.; Gao, H. *Clinical imaging* 2013, *37*, 273–282.

[33] Panetta, K.; Zhou, Y.; Agaian, S.; Jia, H. *Information Technology in Biomedicine, IEEE Transactions on* 2011, *15*, 918–928.

[34] Georgsson, F.; Ols?n, C. The accuracy of geometric approximation of the mamilla in mammograms. In *CARS'03*; 2003.

[35] Haindl, M. *CWI Quarterly* 1991, *4*, 305-331.

[36] Haindl, M. Visual Data Recognition and Modeling Based on Local Markovian Models. In *Mathematical Methods for Signal and Image Analysis and Representation*, Vol. 41; Florack, L.; Duits, R.; Jongbloed, G.; Lieshout, M.-C.; Davies, L., Eds.; Springer London: 2012 10.1007/978-1-4471-2353-8_14.

Chapter 5

Aid System to Evaluation of Breast Calcification by Case-Based Reasoning According to BI-RADS Category

Fatima G.G. Elpidio, Lourdes M. Brasil and Janice M. Lamas

Additional information is available at the end of the chapter

http://dx.doi.org/10.5772/59939

1. Introduction

Breast cancer is a multi-factor disease. It is heterogeneous neoplasm with histopathological changes that has been registered with a high occurrence in women in the last decades according to advance of female age [1].

Early detection and right diagnosis of breast cancer are complex processes that are derived among other factors from reasoning and experience of expert. The Breast Imaging Reporting and Data System (BI-RADS) aims at standardizing mammographic reporting in order to reduce differences in the subjective interpretation of mammographic images and to facilitate the control of the results [2].

Calcifications can be characterized as small radiopaque deposits with high sensitivity to X-rays. Generally, they are associated with benign cases, however they have been found in about 30 to 50% of clinically undetectable lesions [2].

The malignancy level from suspicious breast calcifications can increase or decrease according to their characteristics such as type, size, quantity, and distribution density. Usually have been considered suspicious for malignancy if were grouped and have irregular or linear appearance. Most researchers say that carcinomas are associated with calcification clusters that have more than 5 elements and it are in a larger area than 3 mm from breast [3] [2].

Classifying calcification clusters as benign or malignant is a complex task, often requiring a biopsy (removal process of tissue fragment for microscopic analysis) to do a definitive conclusion. In spite of high probability to diagnose cancer in calcification regions that are suspicious of malignancy [4], researches [5, 12] shows that a amount of problems including false diagnose could be avoided if there was more precise analysis before surgery.

The use of computational techniques on the decision support helps medical professionals to disseminate the implicit knowledge and to map computationally the reasoning processes that lead them to make a decision. In this context, a system of Case-Based Reasoning (CBR) [6] is a computational technique derived from Artificial Intelligence (AI) which uses tacit knowledge to model it into an Expert System able to use previous solutions on case solutions.

The result of this research is also, part of a greater extension project entitled "3D Anatomical Atlas Applied to Breast" with the National Laboratory for Scientific Computing of Rio de Janeiro (NLSC/RJ) that received collaboration between the University of Brasília at Gama (FGA/UNB) and Janice Lamas Clinical Radiology (JLCR).

2. Materials and methods

The system was developed using PHP software language [7], PostgreSQL version 9.0 as relational database and Structured Query Language to access data handling (SQL) [8]. The information requirements for CBR development was done by knowledge elicitation techniques [9] under expert supervision and following similar cases of study. The expert contributed with definition of characteristics and more relevant indices to evaluate the global and local similarity and also to setting the weights for the calculation of the overall similarity. So the main strategies adopted for acquisition and mapping information were as follows:

- *Brainstorming* – It is a technique of meetings where participants suggest and explore ideas [9]. This technique was applied for widely discuss the knowledge domain to the specialist explains the main points that should be considered in problem definition.
- Questionnaires - this approach is useful because it allows to obtain the knowledge in a targeted, practical and concise way. The forms adopted had multiple choice questions, checklist and descriptive questions in order to bunch information on specific topics questions.
- The questionnaires were developed based on lists of importance to the specialist indicates the weights of indices.Interviews – it was followed a script guidelines according to knowledge items that were being analyzed to obtain information efficiently.
- Prototyping - this technique allowed to monitore critical aspects of the requirements, expediting the development and minimizing the risks of system construction [9].

In the end of this step was generated the formal documentation of system requirements and it was defined the scope of the research in order to develop CBR system.

In CBR systems the cases representation can be performed using data directly from the structure where they are or by the generation of a second structure containing only data relevant to the cases composition. The cases representation was done using attribute-value [6] through relationship model entities in table form on relational database [8]. So each case was represented by a record in the table and, consecutively, each field corresponds to a feature of the case. The data were extracted from the database through domain information interpretation, according to methods established by the expert and BI-RADS standard.

These interpretation methods were translated to a computational algorithm to do the cases base automatically. In the cases base algorithm, each instance of case and attribute values were calculated using combinatorics [10] method to appoint the BI-RADS class according to case characteristics. The Figure 1 shows a representation overview of CBR cases structure. The similarity algorithm adopted in CBR system retrieves correlated cases according to characteristics weights and their importance level for BI-RADS classification. Details about analysis of calcifications done by CBR system designed to suggest the BI-RADS classification will be explained at following.

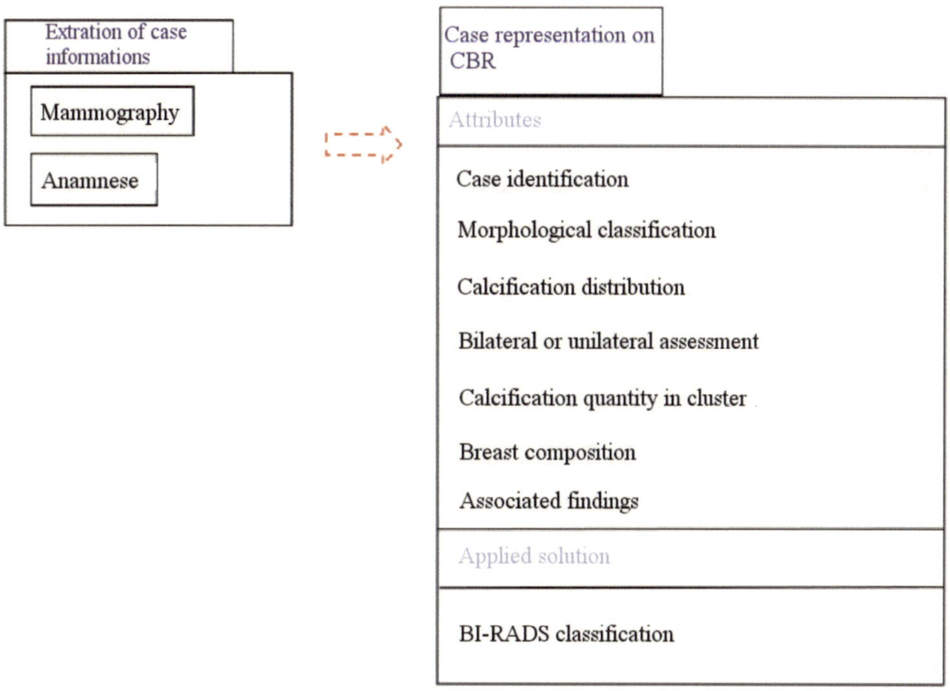

Figure 1. Cases representation structure.

3. Morphology

Breast calcifications are classified in one of those cases BI-RADS described:

- Typically benign if they were skin calcifications, vascular calcifications, coarse or "popcorn-like" calcifications, large rod-like calcifications, round calcifications, lucent-centered calcifications, "eggshell" or "rim" calcifications, milk of calcium calcifications, suture calcifications, dystrophic calcifications.
- Intermediate concern, suspicious calcifications - if they were amorphous or indistinct calcifications or coarse heterogeneous calcifications.
- Higher probability malignancy - if they here fine pleomorphic calcifications, fine linear or fine-linear branching calcifications.

4. Distribution

Distribution modifiers indicate the disposition and consecutive breast calcifications suspicion degree. It was adopted six possibilities proposed by BI-RADS: Diffuse/scattered, Regional, Clustered grouped, Linear or Segmental.

5. Bilateral or unilateral assessment

In general it is considered whether the grouping of calcifications has the same distribution and the same morphology in both mammas, because generally the cases where the features are just one mamma (unilateral) are more associated with suspected malignancy.

6. Breast composition

According to the breast kind, mammography may have a decreased detection sensitivity. The Table 1 describes the possibilities for classification adopted according to BI-RADS.

Breast density	Breast density
The breasts are almost entirely fatty	Glandular tissue <25%
Fibroglandular density	Glandular tissue between 25% and 50%
Heterogeneously dense	Glandular tissue between 51% and 75%
The breasts are extremely dense	Glandular tissue >75%

Table 1. Patterns of breast density by BI-RADS

7. Stability level from calcifications

One way to evaluate the stability of breast calcifications is following previous exams where it is possible to analyze if there was any change in the number of particles, distribution, morphology or associated findings.

8. Calcification quantity in cluster

The reference literature and the expert requirements from area show that above 5 calcifications grouped have a higher degree of suspicion to cancer.

9. Associated findings

They are other structures which may increase the level of malignance suspicion if it were together calcifications. Some associated findings receive a higher priority degree than calcifications for BI-RADS classification. e.g, nodules, focal asymmetry, architectural distortion, etc.

Therefore, BI-RADS class suggestion was done by system based on analysis of the calcification majority found in mammogram using as decision criteria the weight of each risk factor like: breast composition, associated findings, distribution pattern of calcification, bilateral or unilateral assessment, calcification quantity in cluster and the predominant morphological classification which was indicated by Artificial Neural Networks (ANN) specifically, the MultiLayer Perceptron (MLP) [11].

CBR knowledge base had 78,336 cases relating to the classification criteria referenced in the BI-RADS. Beyond this sample, it was used fifty real cases (they came directly from structure), which were used in the validation of the system. The features weight of the represented cases in the CBR system were defined assigning 70% of the weight between the morphology and distribution of calcifications, besides considering if the breast evaluation was bilateral or unilateral. The remaining 30% were distributed between the standard of breast composition, evaluation of particles amount in the calcifications cluster and associated findings.

The similarity measure is a function that measures the similarity between two cases. It is used to define the most similar cases ordering them according to the level of higher similarity. This metric is usually normalized in a range from 0 (total dissimilarity) to 1 (absolute coincidence) and it can be evaluated in a global and local context. Global similarity analyzes the usefulness of a case for a given question, where the similarity between the question and the case should be determined. On the other hand, Local Similarity evaluates similarity in terms of relevant attributes or features of a case. Hence measure of Global similarity adopted by the CBR system was developed using Nearest Neighbor with feature weighting method which it is a technique that determines the nearest neighbor geometrically considering the distance measurement definition and weight (importance degree) for each feature as Equation 1:

$$(T, S) = \sum_{i=1}^{n} SIMi(Ti, Si)^{*}i$$

Where:

a. T is the input case;

b. S is a base case

c. n is attributes quantity of each case;

d. i is a individual attribute-value;

e. SIM is similarity function for the attribute I on T and S cases;

f. weighted nearest neighbor - is the nearest neighbor changed by the weight of the attributes of the case, as expressed in Equation 2.

g. Where w is the weight given to attribute i.

The Step function was adopted to calculate the Local similarity. This method consists in calculating the distance between two values as specified by Equation 2. The result of the local similarity is 1 when the result of the difference is less than the threshold otherwise the result is 0.

$$(vi, vj) = \begin{cases} 1, & ifV(vi - vj)V \leq S \\ 0, & ifV(vi - vj)V > S \end{cases}$$

The Table 2 shows a set of case examples that will be used to explain how the system works during a search execution.

Characteristics	Weight	Case 1	Case 2	Query cases
Morfology	0.35	0	0	0
Distribution	0.35	0.8	0.8	0.8
Bilateral/unilateral assessment	0.02	0.5	0.8	1
Calcification quantity in cluster	0.03	0.2	0.3	0
Breast composition	0.05	0.1	0.1	0.1
Associated findings	0.20	0	0	0

Table 2. Comparing query cases with case bases from CBR system.

http://dx.doi.org/10.5772/59939

Using as an example the case of Table 2 and any query case (C), the calculations performed by algorithm developed to recover the cases of higher similarity with the problem will be explained below. Considering: X=Case 1 and C=Query case. Distance measure between the case X and the query case $C=(0.35*0 - 0 \vee 2)+(0.35*0.8 - 0.8 \vee 2)+(0.02*1 - 0.5 \vee 2)+ (0.03*0 - 0 \vee 2) + (0.05*0.01 - 0.01 \vee 2)+(0.20*0 - 0 \vee 2)1/2$;

Distance measure between the case X and the query case $C = (0.35 * 0) + (0.35 * 0.25) + (0.02 * 1) + (0.03 * 0.04) + (0.05 * 0) + (0.20 * 0)1/2$;

Therefore, the distance measure between the case X and the query case C≈0.33; Considering: X=Case 2 and C=Query case.

Distance measure between the case X and the query case $C = (0.35 * |0 - 0|2) + (0.35 * |0.8 - 0.8|2) + (0.02 * |1 - 0.8|2) + (0.03 * |0 - 0.3|2) + (0.05 * |0.01 - 0.01|2) + (0.20 * |0 - 0|2)1/2$;

Distance measure between the case X and the query case $C = (0.35 * 0) + (0.35 * 0) + (0.02 * 0.04) + (0.03 * 0.09) + (0.05 * 0) + (0.20 * 0)1/2$;

Therefore, the distance measure between the case X and the query case C≈0.06;

According to the calculations made, the most similar case to the new problem is one that has the smallest distance [6]. Therefore, in the example presented the case that has the largest similarity to the query case is Case 2. The attributes used to compare the similarity between input cases and the case bases was done using explanation technique according to expert requirements. Because despite the existence of several methods for automatic cases indexing, the researches shows that the best strategy is still the choice of manual indexes, as adopted in this work.

The recovery of similarity measure between cases is calculated sequentially for all the case bases in order to determining the x most similar cases. Search by global similarity between new cases related to previous cases inserted at the base is done using the nearest neighbor algorithm weighted normalized besides metrics for measuring contrast. Storage of new cases is done manually, so it is necessary human intervention to register new cases in the system. In each case of base is analyzed successively the ratio of specific preference for the situation by measures of similarity of the system. All cases of the base are arranged according to the result of the similarity function. The local similarities set was calculated for each case attribute using the standard BI-RADS applied in a staircase function.

In this work it was chosed the zero adjustment, which is generally used in situations of complex problems, but with simple solutions. As discussed previously, the tacit reasoning involved to distinguish benign calcifications of suspected malignancy is a complex process, however the resolution applied in the scope of this proposal is a bit simple: it consist in to indicate the BI-RADS category most applicable based on risk factors referenced in the literature.

The solution evaluation was performed by an expert, in addition, we adopted the technique of predictive validation [2] using the concepts of sensitivity and specificity used with historical cases in known diagnostic tests. The Figure 2 summarizes the reasoning structure adopted in the CBR functional components scope.

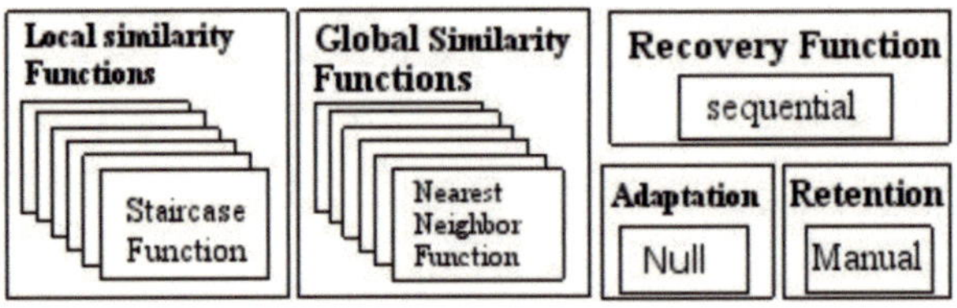

Figure 2. Reasoning Structure adopted in this research.

10. Results

So if a query is done in system developed which has X number of cases, it shows an electronic form to be filled with important characteristics from risk factor to cancer diagnosis.

The system conducts a search by measure of contrast and returns a set of cases where it is applied to the nearest neighbor algorithm to show the most applicable BI-RADS class according to the solution of similar previous cases present in the CBR database system.

The following figures show system interfaces with its steps to recover similarity cases.

The Figure 3 shows the system interface used to do a searching in its database.

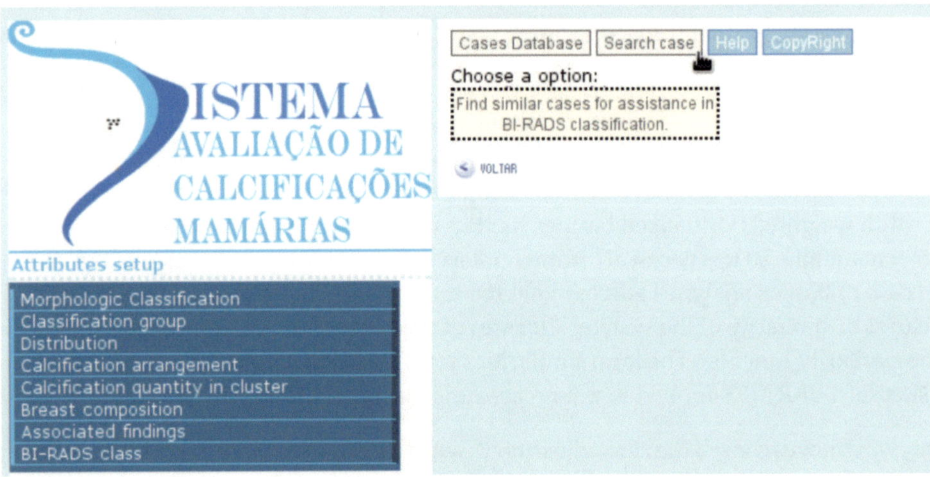

Figure 3. System interface to access the option for query cases.

The Figure 4 shows the system interface to fill characteristics of case searched.

This screen allows a similarity search in the RBC system by fill in a form with the calcification risk factors previously described. After it to fill feature of query case the CBR developed performs a similarity search based in its base cases and shows a suggestion of

BI-RADS class as illustrated Figure 5.

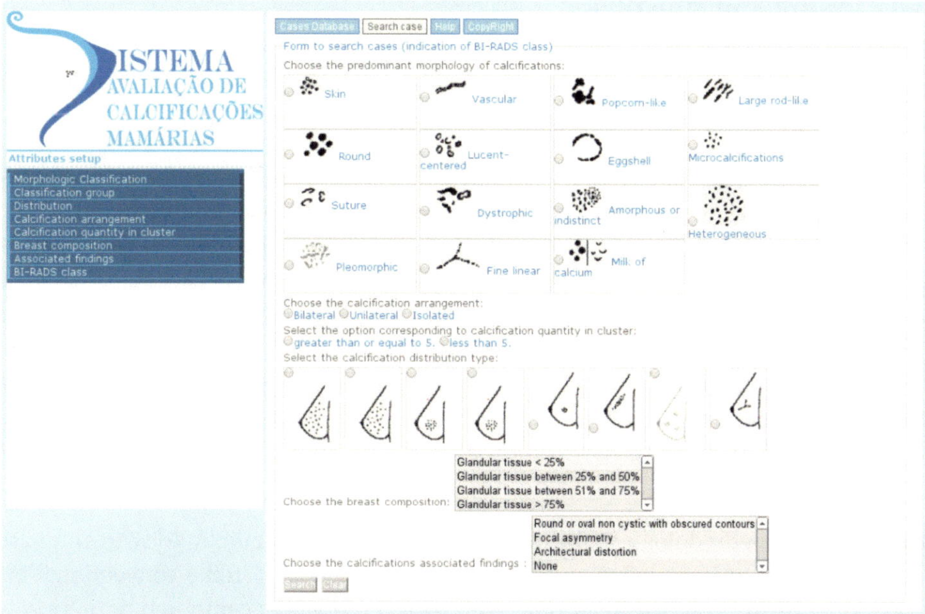

Figure 4. Search form used in CBR system.

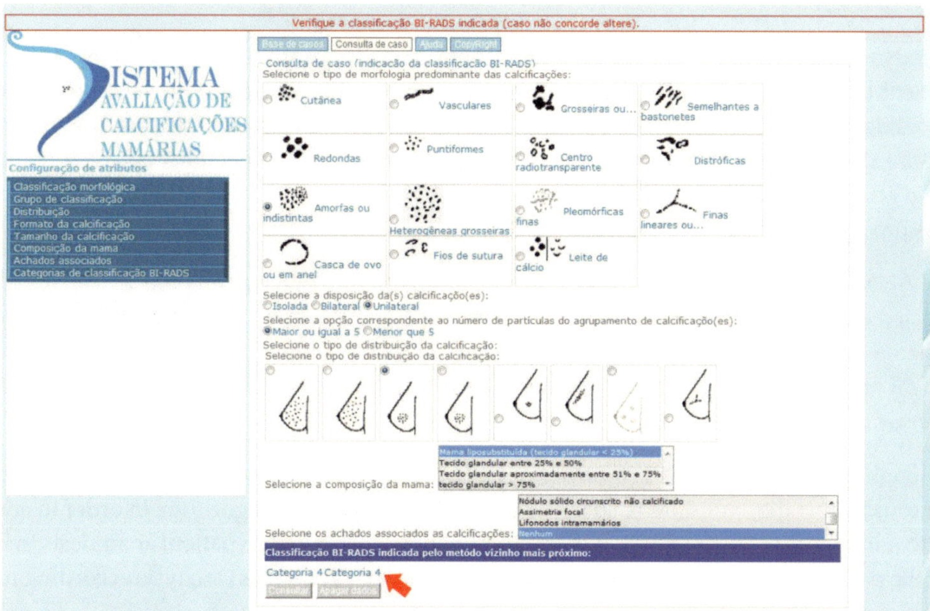

Figure 5. interface of CBR developed that shows the BI-RADS class based on features of case query.

11. Discussion and conclusion

Both ANNs as CBR are AI techniques of enshrined in the acquisition and utilization of information to generate solutions similar to human reasoning in specialized fields.

In general, the ANN is an alternative to the traditional computing model based on the model of Von Neumann Machines. They are proven effective in solving computational problems, such as learning by examples or patterns of input data, whose main line of resolution is the inference rules of entry set to absorb the learning and consecutively reaching generalization of knowledge. The ANNs also differ from conventional programming by not requiring explicit programming. They do not adopt the paradigm of imperative programming, they use the connectionist paradigm which learns by examples using the analogy of solving problems based on previous solutions. Another ANN's advantage is their ability to test all possible reactions to parallel stimuli and their generalization ability if there are incompleteness of the data presented for the problem.

Whereas the CBR methodology characterizes the paradigm of symbolic AI with emphasis on mathematical logic to knowledge representation at high level. Unlike conventional expert systems using the Rules Based Reasoning with logical sequences composed of premises and conclusions, CBR modeling knowledge from a database of cases that constitute the knowledge previously experienced. Usually each case has a problem description and its solution, which may contain a set of successes and failures related cases resolved. CBR case base uses inferences strategies to identify the current situation and find a similar experience on its memory to solve a new problem.

The advantage of using a hybrid system, although in different tasks, is to expand and complement the potential of each approach. If on one hand the ANNs are powerful tools in the knowledge acquisition for other way they have difficulties to explain the proposed solution because they are as a "black-box" which maps the weight of connections between neurons. But in general, CBR besides to map the knowledge by its cases base, it is able to show the way of its process decision.

The ANN MPL adopted indicated the predominant morphological type of calcifications detected on mammography. However, for effective analysis in order to establish a diagnosis of mammography, it is necessary a complete analysis also reviewing the patient's anamnese. So CBR and ANN were adopted together to assist in the analysis and BI-RADS classification of breast calcification.

Although there are some solid solutions of CBR, the most of them has some restrictions of use that could affect the experiment, so it was decided to develop the algorithm, in order to ensure the requirements of this research. It was filtered the risk factors from patient anamnesis to keep just the parameters that has higher importance in breast calcification analysis according to BI-RADS.

One of the problems faced in breast calcifications system developing was that, in general, the BI-RADS protocol says that the radiologist should describe in his mammography report just

http://dx.doi.org/10.5772/59939

the greater suspicions found or those that may raise doubts by other professional interpretations. However, this proposal performs an independent assessment of suspicion level from breast calcifications. Hence there was difficulty in collecting information about typically benign calcifications, which are usually not referenced in the reports because they have a low degree of suspicion. So combinatorics technique was used based on indices analyzed in order to generate the CBR base case and to cover these situations creating a broad enough base, covering all possible cases under expert orientation and BI-RADS protocol.

For while the calcifications stability level is not used by CBR developed, but on next CBR algorithm versions it will be increase this parameter, which also has great relevance in the analysis of breast calcifications.

This proposal was done to provide a system for aiding the evaluation of breast calcifications. With the methodology and results is possible to validate that this proposal provides a consistent process for analyzing breast calcifications that can be used like a second opinion to the experts.

Author details

Fatima G.G. Elpidio[1*], Lourdes M. Brasil[1] and Janice M. Lamas[2]

*Address all correspondence to: fgizele@hotmail.com

1 University of Brasília at Gama (UnB /FGA) / Post-Graduation Program in Biomedical Engineering, Gama, Brazil

2 Janice Lamas Radiology Clinic, Brazil

References

[1] WHO. Breast Cancer. http://www.who.int Accessed 2014-04-07.

[2] A.C.R: Breast Imaging Reporting and Data System (BI-RADS), 3rd edn. American College of Radiology, VA (2003).

[3] Martins, L.A.L., Barra, A.A., Lucena, C.E.M.: Microcalcificacoes mamárias suspeitas de malignidade. Revista Brasileira de Cancerologia 27(3), 262–6 (2006).

[4] Kouskos, E.e.a.: Wire localisation biopsy of non-palpable breast lesions: reasons of unsuccessful excision. Eur J Gynaecol Oncol 27(3), 262–6 (2006).

[5] Biffi, R.G.: A dinâmica familiar de um grupo de mulheres com câncer de mama. Tese de doutorado. PhD thesis, Escola de Enfermagem de Ribeirão Preto, USP (2003).

[6] Michael, M.R., Weber, R.O.: Case-Based Reasoning. A Textbook, 1st ed. Springer, New York (2013).

[7] Reiersol, D., Baker, M., Shiflett, C.: PHP in Action: Objects, Design, Agility., 1st ed. Manning Publications Co, Greenwich, Conn (2007).

[8] Date, C.J.: Database Design and Relational Theory, 1st ed. O'Reilly Media, CA (2012).

[9] Pressman, R. S. Software engineering: a practitioner's approach, McGraw-Hill Higher Education, 2010.

[10] Brualdi, R.A.: Introduction to Combinatorics, 5th ed. Pearson, New York (2009).

[11] Elpídio, F.G.G., et al: Artificial neural network to classify breast calcification in accordance with morphological analysis described by birads and le gal (in portuguese: Classificação de calcificações mamárias baseado na análise morfológica descrita por birads e le gal através de rede neural artificial). In: XXIII Congresso Brasileiro de Engenharia Biomedica (2012).

[12] Elpidio, F.G.G. Aid System to Evaluation of Breast Calcification by Digital Processing of Images and Artificial Intelligence (in portuguese: Sistema de Auxílio na Avaliação de Calcificações Mamárias por Processamento Digital de Imagens e Inteligência Artificial), RIUnB, 2012.

Chapter 6

Availability of Mammographs in Brazil

Cleber da Silva Alves,
Marília Miranda Forte Gomes and
Lourdes Mattos Brasil

Additional information is available at the end of the chapter

http://dx.doi.org/10.5772/60792

1. Introduction

The Brazilian Constitution ensures in Article 196 that health is a right of every citizen and duty of the State, guaranteed through social and economic policies aimed at reducing the risk of illness and other hazards and the universal and equal access to actions and services for their promotion, protection and recovery [1]. Under the legal aspect, there is no distinction between social and economic groups, and especially concerning pathologies. This assertion is reaffirmed by Law 8080 of 1990 (Organic Law of Health) where health is declared as a fundamental human right, imposing on the State the duty to provide the necessary conditions to its full enjoyment by the preparation and implementation of economic and social policies aimed at reducing the risks of diseases and other hazards and at establishing conditions that ensure universal and equal access to actions and services for their promotion, protection and recovery [2].

As noted, the State has undertaken to draw up policies for the prevention and treatment of diseases of epidemiological interest. To be successful in such endeavor, it is therefore necessary to examine the country in its epidemiological and demographic context, so that, we can scale where there are greater demands for health care for the population. It is worth mentioning that Brazil is undergoing a profound demographic transition caused mainly by the decline in fertility that began in the mid 60s and widespread in all Brazilian regions and social strata [3].

From this perspective, it appears that the magnitude of the increase in demand for health care grows with the aging population. Taking into account this measure of population growth, there has been a considerable increase in the incidence of chronic non-communicable diseases (NCDs), becoming the largest global health problem and relating directly to the high number of premature deaths, loss of quality of life, with high degree of limitation and disability as well as economic impacts on families, communities and society in general [4].

Estimates indicate that between 75-80% of the population at the age of 60 and over have at least one chronic condition, resulting in a contingent of 27 million in 2025 and 50 million in 2050. A similar up-scaling exercise, considering the disability, would result, in 2025, in 6.7 million older people with inevitable necessity of care and medical attention, and 12 million in 2050 [3].

Another important issue that can not be ignored, is that the development of a chronic disease in an individual of working age brings social and economic consequences since there is a decrease in productive capacity and also contributes to the increase in demand for health services. In Brazil, as in other countries, NCDs also consist of the health problem of greater magnitude and correspond to 72% of the causes of death, particularly for diseases of the circulatory system (31.3%), cancer (16.3 %), diabetes (5.2%) and chronic respiratory disease (5.8%) [4, 5].

In the wake of these considerations, it is important to note that breast cancer has too much importance in the epidemiological context of the country, because it is the type of cancer that affects more women around the world, including Brazil [6]. Mortality from breast cancer was the fifth leading cause of death for women between the ages of 30 to 39 years in Brazil and the third leading cause of death for women between the ages of 40 to 49 years. The specific rate of mortality from breast cancer for women between the ages of 40 to 49 years old was 17.2 deaths per 100,000 women [7]. In 2014, there is a prediction that occur 57,120 new cases of breast cancer in the country [8], and the increased incidence of the disease is accompanied by increased mortality, which can be mainly attributed to a delay in diagnosis and of appropriate therapy implementation [9].

Taking the limitations of the Brazilian public healthcare system, the rapid aging process points to the need to redefine the policies of this sector in order to prevent, or at least mitigate, the helpless population [3]. Still, one cannot overlook that the secondary prevention of breast cancer is based on early detection through screening of asymptomatic women and, therefore, the Ministry of Health recommends mammography every two years for women between 50 to 69 years old [7, 10]. Notwithstanding the policy proposed by the federal government to prevent breast cancer, studies have shown that there is a prevalence of women in the country who, throughout life, never had a mammogram performed both in the youngest age group (46%) and in older (49%) [11] showing that only the adoption of a policy for the prevention of disease is not enough to reach the population.

A radical shift in demand consequent to the changing age structure of the population requires the upgrading of the health system in aspects of infrastructure and human resources, as well as the development of extensive technical and methodological basis which includes a review of procedures and care protocols [3], in particular those that may contribute to the increased availability of existing mammography equipment in the country.

http://dx.doi.org/10.5772/60792

2. Problem statement

A study from 2010 stated that mammography devices acquired with public resources could cover, if rightly managed, the entire population of users in the country, however they only comply with 15 to 20% of that population. The low number of mammograms performed did not cover 20% of the equipment installed capacity [12]. From this premise it is evident the necessity of extending management actions on equipment to obtain better results within the population scope. In this regard, the National Congress of Brazil, after conducting debate on issues concerning the use of public resources in the acquisition of mammography devices and preventive detection of breast cancer, revealed through information obtained from experts in the field, that the devices were not being fully used and that early diagnosis were not being made in sufficient number. Based on these assumptions, the Congress requested the Federal Audit Court (TCU) to verify the application of federal funds in the acquisition, control and maintenance of mammography in the public health system, the private system and network of accredited units [13].

In response to the request made by the National Congress was determined to conduct a nationwide audit to diagnose the causes of low productivity of mammograms for the Brazilian population.

Already in the audit planning phase, through a cause and effect analysis factors that could possibly contribute to the limitation of performing mammograms were identified. The problems highlighted were grouped into six categories: devices, low number of mammogram requests, structure of health facilities, inputs, professionals and increased demand. These categories were then subdivided in accordance with the nature of core problems, and then grouped and arranged in a diagrammatic form shown in Figure 1.

The diagram prepared by TCU is a graphic tool in which the causes of the problem were represented by arrows, gathered to represent the effects they cause one another until their peak at the problem analysis. As can be seen, the possible causes which, together, contribute to non-attainment of mammography screening in women aged above 50 years are from diverse backgrounds, highlighting the multidisciplinary character necessary to achieve a solution, or at least minimize their effects.

To the Court of Audits, the root causes of the problem are as follows:

1. Equipment

1.1. Inadequate geographic allocation

1.1.1. Inadequacy/noncompliance with the PDR

1.1.2. Technical opinion issued contrary to the parameters

1.1.3. Inadequate technical recommendation

1.1.4. Deficiency in CNES

1.1.5. Requests without technical considerations

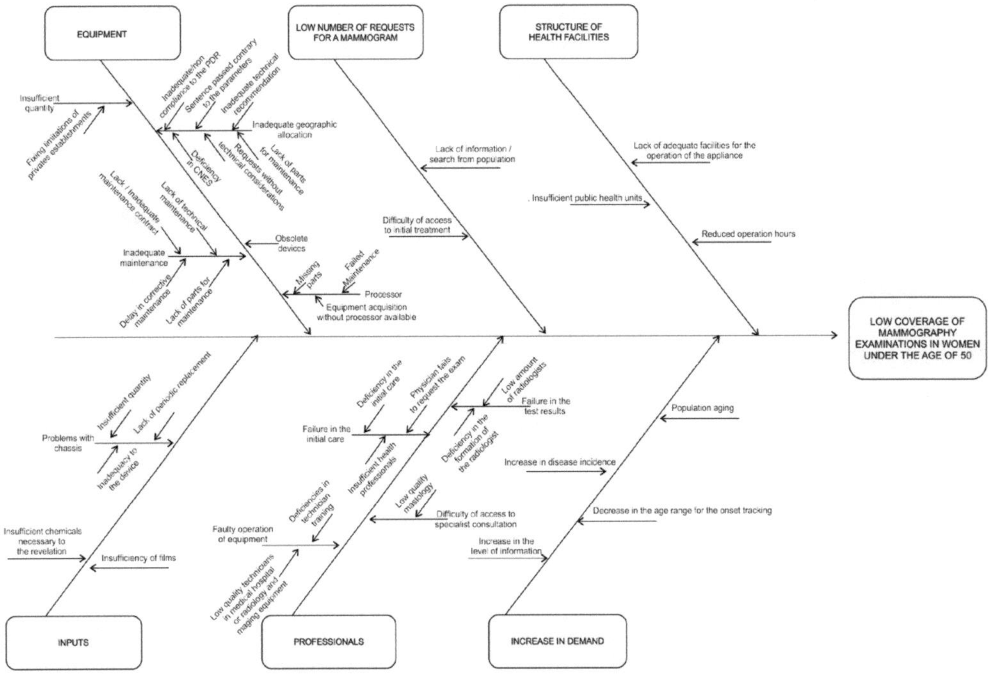

Figure 1. Limiting factors for mammography. Source: Adapted from ACORDAO nº 247/2010 – TCU – Plenário

1.1.6. Insufficient private facilities

1.2. Insufficient quantity

1.2.1. Setting forth of limitations for private facilities

1.3. Inadequate maintenance

1.3.1. Lack of maintenance technicians

1.3.2. Lack / Inadequate maintenance contract

1.3.3. Delay in corrective maintenance

1.3.4. Lack of maintenance parts

1.4. Obsolete devices

1.5. Processor

1.5.1. Lack of parts

1.5.2. Failed Maintenance

1.5.3. Equipment acquisition without processor available

2. Low number of requests for a mammogram

2.1. Lack of information / search by the population

2.2. Difficulty of access to initial treatment

3. Structure of health facilities

3.1. Lack of adequate facilities for device operation

3.2. Insufficient public health units

3.3. Reduced operation hours

4. Inputs

4.1. Insufficiency of films

4.2. Insufficient chemicals necessary for the development

4.3. Problems with chassis

4.3.1. Insufficient quantity

4.3.2. Lack of periodic replacement

4.3.3. Inadequacy to the device

5. Professionals

5.1. Difficulty of access to specialist consultation

5.1.1. Low quality mastologists

5.2. Failure in the test results

5.2.1 Deficiency in the qualification of the radiologist

5.2.2. Low amount of radiologists

5.3. Failure in the initial care

5.3.1. Deficiency in the initial care

5.3.2. Physician fails to request the exam

5.3.3. Insufficient health professionals

5.4. Faulty operation of equipment

5.4.1. Deficiencies in technician training

5.4.2. Low quality technicians in medical hospital or radiology and imaging equipment

6. Increase in demand

6.1. Increase in disease incidence

6.2. Population aging

6.3. Increase in the information level

6.4. Decrease in the age range for the onset tracking

The audit report of the TCU showed that after the survey through questionnaires sent to health organizations selected for sampling among the six categories of root causes, three stood out by the amount of replies of healthcare facilities queried, pointing a number of flaws that interfere with the way it offers tests for the target audience. The emphasis was given to the inputs, and maintenance professionals, the latter being that concentrating the largest number of events reported by health facilities (Figure 2).

Considering the information gathered in the TCU report, the maintenance of mammography devices and development equipment is the main factor that leads to reduction or interruption of mammography, becoming a serious and frequent problem. It is observed that often there is difficulty on the part of health facilities in acquiring parts for maintenance as well as difficulties in hiring technicians to perform the services.

The TCU analysis further points that regarding the group of factors related to maintenance, were verified problems related to lack of maintenance contract, delay on part replacement, deficiency of maintenance services and processor defects [13].

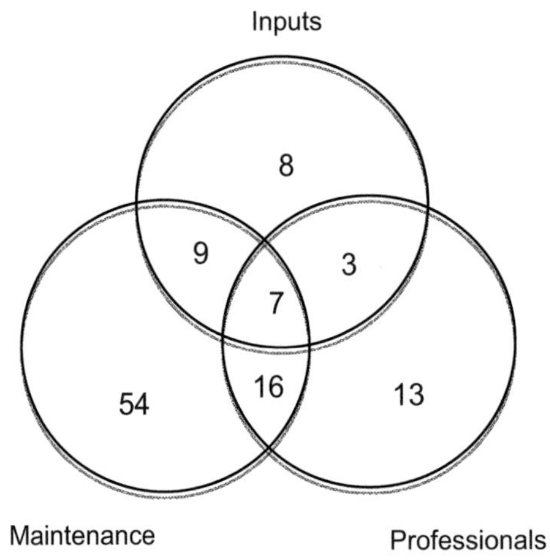

Figure 2. Venn-Euler Diagram: Limiting factors for mammograms. Source: Adapted from ACÓRDÃO nº 247/2010 – TCU – Plenário

As a result of lack of equipment maintenance, it was reported the existence of mammography device stopped for two years because of lack of spare parts for the old and outdated processors, without the possibility of performing maintenance and acquisition of spare parts. It has also been reported that when the obsolete processors worked, the films went out wet and the drying process was performed by means of improvised hanging lines. Some facilities reported having mammography device that had never worked because the acquisition of the mammography device was not associated with the acquisition of processor or indication how could the exams development be performed [13].

In regard to the physical infrastructure involving room shielding, refrigeration, construction or renovation works, electrical and plumbing installation, the TCU report indicates that equipment are purchased without the necessary planning related to the physical infrastructure for the equipment to be installed and its operation after delivery by the supplier. In addition, there are health centers that inform lack of sufficiency for electricity supply to the hospital, which might cause damage to the equipment during the usage phase [13].

One cannot overlook the importance of infrastructure for equipment allocation. The report notes that in a considerable amount of health units, the mammography devices acquired never became operational due to problems of structure and inadequate room shielding where the mammography device would be installed, an inadequate cooling system, need for construction works of the physical space or renovation of the existing one, inadequate electrical installations, and inadequate plumbing system. Being common for some facilities to concentrate more than one of these inadequacies.

As far as the TCU is concerned, these limitations (together or separately) resulted, to some extent, in disruption of mammography services in health facilities, poor quality of images generated, reducing the number of periods of service to the population, as well as delay in the deadline for submission of exam reports. In these conditions, retired devices are under deterioration and loss of the warranty term by lapse of time without being used.

In the country, the decisions to purchase medical equipment for health facilities are often taken with respect to a sector/department or isolated event, without giving them a multi-departmental emphasis. It is observed that, generally, the major concern of managers is focused on the acquisition and execution of works and procurement of equipment, without planning the use, maintenance and supplies [13,14]. There are reports of cases where health services eventually receive medical equipment without being in the least aware of their purchase with no prediction of qualified personnel, infrastructure and supplies to keep the device in operation [13].

Such assertions demonstrate the fact of the need to schedule the acquisition of certain equipment with the necessary infrastructure to operate it in order to provide greater availability of equipment and full use of its production capacity. In this context, actually concerning the mammography equipment purchased in the country, there is a decoupling of investment planning in the purchase of mammography equipment and further financing of production costs, without consideration at the time of the incorporation of this technology, the cost stipulated for the operation [13]. As far as the TCU is concerned, equipment is acquired without taking into consideration the necessary logistical support such as hiring of administrative and technical staff, purchase of supplies and hiring of maintenance.

Despite the clear need to implement maintenance plans, both preventive and corrective, as well as the benefits arising from them, limiting factors such as insufficient material, financial, and human resources restrict the development of these programs, especially in Brazil and, particularly, in the service public [14,15].

Another important decision to be made by the local health manager refers to the place of maintenance of the equipment, which can occur both internally - within the institution itself - as being contracted externally, especially for those equipment with the most electronic complexity. Such decisions should be based both on the availability of material and human resources as the costs for training and maintenance of specialized personnel. In this sense, it is important that managers consider the following factors: 1) the existence of trained personnel for maintenance of every type and model of equipment; 2) existence of technical documentation relating to the equipment to receive internal maintenance; 3) existence of test and calibration equipment for the evaluation of equipment after maintenance as some types of equipment, particularly those that represent risks to the patient, require security and/or calibration tests after a preventive or corrective maintenance; 4) proximity of the manufacturer/ technical representative of the equipment; and 5) the possibility of acquiring original [14] pieces.

The GM/MS Ordinance No. 1101, of June 12, 2002, establishes the parameters of health care coverage under the Unified Health System (SUS) and sets forth in its item 2.7.2, the coverage of a mammography device for every 240,000 inhabitants. At the same time, the National Cancer Institute (INCA), through technical note, has established as a production parameter of a mammography device, 6,758 mammograms/year, obtained as follows: 32 examinations /day x 22 working days/month x 12 months x 80% production capacity = 6758 mammograms/year.

Asked about the reason to establish that an equipment should produce 80% of its capacity (at the possibility of producing 100%), INCA reported that:

To calculate the capacity of a mammography device, INCA held that a professional can perform a mammogram every 15 minutes or 4 mammograms/hour, such information is obtained from professionals who perform the exam. This analysis considered only the use of a simple mammography device.

Assuming an 8-hour shift for 22 days in the month, it would be possible to perform 704 mammograms/month.

During the year would be possible to perform 8,448 mammograms/year. However, assessing that actually a device does not use 100% of its capacity, since during the year there are holidays, vacations of the professional who performs the examination, technical problems related to equipment and its maintenance, it was estimated that this "downtime" would be about 20%.

We emphasize that this parameter was built for a simple-type mammography device and that the production capacity must serve to guide the use of the equipment and should not restrict its operation, once it is locally evaluated that it is possible to go beyond it [17].

What is observed is that the INCA itself identifies two impediments for achieving the fullness of equipment operation, and maintenance personnel. Therefore, it is observed that if the equipment can provide adequate maintenance, it would also be possible to expand the examination production capacity by mammography equipment.

3. Application area

In the wake of TCU considerations, this case study was developed with the goal of showing among the root causes listed by TCU, which can primarily be handled by the clinical engineering department of the health organization because the problems pointed out transcend several professional categories. Thus, this paper focuses dealing with those issues relating to the responsibilities of the clinical engineer, as defined by the American College of Clinical Engineering (ACCE), namely: a Clinical Engineer is a professional who supports and advances patient care by applying engineering and managerial skills to healthcare technology [16].

The Clinical Engineering relates directly to what is most modern and efficient in the management of medical-hospital technologies. Taking into consideration the developmental stage reached by the science of Biomedical Engineering, associated with the increasing level of complexity of modern hospital equipment and facilities, as well as the costs involved in their acquisition and maintenance there is an increasing need of highly qualified professional training to relate to this technology to make the most of their productive capacity and increased availability. For that it is necessary that these professionals know the whole life cycle of equipment and technologies, thus being able to perform the necessary actions in order to achieve the best results with the patient.

The speed of development of new technologies is important to the clinical engineer concerning the participation in decision making processes of incorporating technologies since this professional is able to mediate the dialogue between health professionals and engineering providing crucial information for decision making regarding the selection between various emerging technologies and the infrastructure needed to support him/her. Thus, the areas of technical and scientific knowledge that should compose the list of skills of the clinical engineer pervade areas such as electrical, electronic, mechanical, civil engineering, biomedicine, sanitation, medical biology, health technologies, state of the specialized market, capacity to perform analyzes, issuance of technical opinions, drafting and project management, and training of health professionals.

The case study prepared involved a health unit with features of a large general hospital, located in the city of Brasília. An analysis of the limiting factors in the report of the TCU that can be treated by Clinical Engineering of the hospital unit was held as part of this health facility. It is worth noting that even some aspects that relate to the equipment are highly dependent on a policy for the sector, which may be the subject of further study.

4. Method used

From the reflection of the problems highlighted by the availability of equipment and mammography, were selected for analysis in this paper, the problems related to the equipment and its processors:

a. Mammogram devices: inadequate technical recommendation, requests without technical considerations, inadequate maintenance, lack of maintenance technicians, lack/inadequacy of the maintenance contract, delay in corrective maintenance, delay in maintenance and lack of spare parts for obsolete equipment.

b. Processor: lack of parts, failure to maintain and purchase equipment without processor available.

Aiming to analyze in field how the processes favoring the increased availability of equipment occur, such as maintenance, a case study was conducted in a general hospital located in the city of Brasília. The hospital was opened in 1972 and has in its radiology unit facilities for providing diagnostics with equipment such as MRI, CT scanner, Pet Scan, Gamma Camera, Hemodynamics, densitometer and remote-controlled RX. The health unit concerned has in its structure a department of education and research that undertakes to provide training and education to their employees and still provides support for foreign researchers with respect to the provision of necessary permits to conduct research within the scope of the organization beyond the Research Ethics Committee (CEP). Regarding the management of medical equipment, the health unit has a contract with a company of clinical engineering, qualified to provide technical assistance on less complex equipment and also to provide advice with respect to equipment that require hiring with specialized suppliers as is the case of mammography devices.

The field research sought to investigate from multiple sources of evidence the organization of health care in the phenomenon of availability of mammography equipment. The case study concerned sought to correlate the procedures performed by the health unit with those prescribed by both the National Health Surveillance Agency (RDC 2, 2010) as prescribed by the Brazilian Association of Technical Standards through ABNT NBR 15943: 2011 - Guidelines for a management program of health service infrastructure equipment and health equipment [18].

The standard was selected because it provides minimum components required for the implementation of an equipment management plan to provide their higher availability and minimize the risks arising from the use of health technologies. The standard was designed to be applied to health services as well as companies that provide management of equipment for health services or still provide logistical support services to health services.

Another relevant aspect of the selected norm for the case study is that it specifies the minimum guidelines that involve the management of technologies such as structuring the documentation to be produced during the life cycle of the equipment, as well as the need to allocate resources in order to manage such technologies.

For the analysis of the hospital organization, the norm concerned provided a number of standard procedures where it was possible to observe its organization structure, infrastructure, personnel management, documentation management, specific requirements applied to the management of mammography, such as planning and selection, purchasing, receiving, verification and acceptance, procedure for the acceptance testing of the equipment, installation, equipment history log and archiving, training, usage, technical intervention, decommissioning and disposal and recording of adverse events related to the equipment.

The methodology selected for the analysis was the case study, which represented a way to capture the differences among the studied health units with that configuration common to the healthcare organizations surveyed by TCU [19].

The case study, of single case, the way it was conducted was described by Yin as a logical way to analyze an element that represents a critical case in testing a well-formulated theory. The theory must specify a clear set of propositions, as well as the circumstances under which the propositions are supposed to be true [20].

Upon confirming, contesting or extending the theory, there must be a unique case satisfying all conditions to test the theory. The only case can then be used to determine whether the propositions of a theory is correct or if some other set of alternative explanations may be more relevant.

Considering the need to collect data directly in the health unit under analysis, the research had characteristics of a field study involving descriptive and exploratory aspects. The descriptive aspects consisted in empirical research whose primary purpose was the design and analysis of the characteristics of the health service and evaluation of internal processes adopted culminating with the possibility of increased availability of mammography equipment.

Regarding the exploratory characteristics, these were evidenced in the research itself, performed in the field, on the premises of the health unit. The aim was to formulate questions with employees of the health unit, with three purposes: developing hypotheses, increasing the familiarity of the researcher with the environment, and also clarifying of theoretical concepts. The study methodology was appropriate for the research, because when entering the halls of the health unit to conduct the research, it was possible to understand environmental issues such as organizational structure available, forms of interaction among units and how the hierarchy of the processes described in the study was established.

Delimitation of the study: a case study of single case, exploratory-descriptive nature combined, performed in a hospital located in the city of Brasília, DF, classified as a general hospital, financed by public funds from the Union on the management of mammography devices on the basis of ANVISA RDC No. 2 of 2010 [21] and ABNT NBR 15943: 2011. The selection criteria of the sample was a non-probabilistic, purposive sampling, with the election of a hospital located in the city of Brasília, DF.

For the research purposes, this type of sampling was efficient, where was up to the researcher, to deal appropriately with his/her limitations, in order to provide the best way to replicate the study in other health units of the same size and specifications without disregard those factors that impose special conditions for replication, such as environmental, social, cultural ones.

5. Results

The health service in response to the determination of the National Health Surveillance Agency (ANVISA) implemented in its unit a Plan of Management Technologies in Health, as determined by RDC 2, of 2010 of ANVISA. In this sense, a firm of clinical engineering specialized in creating and implementing the referred plan was hired, acting as consultant of the Hospital Board in issues related to the acquisition and incorporation of new technologies. For a perfect execution of the procedures, a contract, which sets out the rights and duties of both parties, indicators to measure the quality of services, provided and the payment, was signed between the service provider and the hospital. If the contracted party does not reach the quality level desired and stated in the contract, there is on the part of the health care organization, ways to decrease the amount to be paid, so that the service provider receives as per delivered quality.

The contract signed with the clinical engineering company aims to establish minimum actions regarding care for the health technologies through management actions and advisory services or specialized consulting. Thus, the institution aims to meet what is being set forth by Resolution RDC No. 2 of ANVISA, in order to ensure the implementation of measures to ensure traceability, quality, efficacy, effectiveness and safety of health technologies.

Among the actions enforced by the contract, there is a focus on management (i.e. receipt, alienation /disposal, installation, uninstallation and operability.), corrective and preventive maintenance, calibration and specialized consulting in technology (infrastructure and equipment).

Therefore, it is intended to achieve on a continuous and sustainable basis the quality of care for the treatment and hospitalization of the target audience of health institution, requiring general and specialized medical and surgical treatment. Another aspect to be considered is to optimize the application of resources for the maintenance and use of the technology park, aiming to achieve excellence in the management of medical-hospital equipment, increase in safety and reliability of medical equipment, their facilities, infrastructure and quality of care.

In order to reach the expected results with the hiring company, the hospital unit undertook to technically qualify the company that should execute the contract. For that, the technical issues that should be covered by the company were incorporated into the contract:

Registration of the company, with the Regional Council of Engineering and Architecture (CREA), in the areas of electrical, mechanical and civil engineering (or architecture), indicated by the technician responsible for the contract performance.

Requirement that the company have in its staff, an engineer with postgraduation (specialization, masters or PhD) in Biomedical Engineering or Clinical Engineering to supervise the activities of the company, other than the Registration of Technical Responsibility (ART) for services object of the present specifications, on behalf of the engineer qualified for this purpose, belonging to the permanent technical staff of the company.

Activities of equipment management are the responsibility of a public servant appointed by the Director of the Health Unit as a contract manager with the outsourced company. His/her professional duties and responsibilities are formally described (in the mammography device maintenance contract), which provides this servant with the capacity to engage with the work to be done on a supported basis by the organization.

For these professionals, trainings that involve the knowledge of management actions including knowledge of the law applied to the issue are performed. The trainings are conducted by a dedicated department, and the content taught is directed as activities developed by professionals with a record of their achievement and participation of these professionals.

The clinical engineering company hired to manage the technology park keeps writing record of the activities described in the Plan of Technology Management in Health with all Standard Operating Procedures (POPs) described and approved by the contract manager.

With regards to the mechanisms established by the health service to generate, store and make available technical and managerial information about the equipment and the procedures used by the health service, there is a systematic documented and enforced by the people in charge, safeguarding that all records are performed manually in books and other paper documents. These records document all the events related to incidents and equipment failures, technical calls, scheduled visits of technicians in equipment maintenance, procedures, replacement of parts or pieces of equipment. All activities recorded in the books and documents are signed and dated by those who performed the procedure.

In the radiology unit, all of mammography documentation, including their manuals, manufacturer´s guidelines, record of calibrations and procedures performed at the frequency established by the equipment manufacturer are grouped and stored.

The resources required to implement the planning of technology management, derive from a budget planning prepared by the management of the hospital organization, taking into account the balance between the needs of the unit and resources availability provided by the Union.

The health unit had until then in its premises an analog mammography equipment and effected its technological upgrading to a digital equipment. Feasibility studies were completed, taking into account the demand for mammography, production capacity of the equipment, resources required for incorporation of the digital equipment, as well as the need to adapt to the existing machine to accommodate the new environment without compromising provision of services to the population served.

In the selection phase of the technology to be incorporated, the health service established technical criteria to be met by potential suppliers candidates to sell the equipment. The prominence given by the health unit refers to the regularity of both the equipment as its suppliers with the body of sanitary control of the country, as well as with the validity of the importation (if it were produced in the country) of all parts of the equipment.

The procurement of equipment is performed by a bidding process complying with the provisions of Law 8,666 dated June 21, 1993 [22]. The hospital maintains a purchase unit by bidding procedure, in which all processes and procedures related to the procurement are recorded. Further, in compliance with the procurement legislation, all acts are published in the official union gazette, thus giving transparency as regards the spending of public funds.

After the procurement procedures, already during the receipt of the equipment, the health service has established criteria for receiving equipment involving analysis: (1) of the technical specifications of the equipment (comparison between what is being delivered with what has been specified for acquisition); (2) regarding evidence of the regularization of equipment with ANVISA; (3) tax documents and other manuals (required to be written in the vernacular language).

The stage of receipt and acceptance of mammography comprises: (1) receipt of the equipment parts in a box (health unit); (2) opening and checking of contents of the boxes (supplier); (3) installation of equipment (supplier); (4) checking of specifications (provider and health unit); (5) acceptance testing (supplier and health unit), and (6) training of users (provider and health unit). All stages of receipt are documented, signed and dated by the participating parties.

The installation of mammography device involved analysis of the infrastructure recommended both by the manufacturer as health monitoring and nuclear energy bodies. Testing and equipment acceptance procedures involve tests that must be met. If during the tests and trials phase nonconformities are detected with the object originally described, the equipment should be listed as unfit for use until the inconsistency has not been remedied.

The acceptance tests are formalized in the mammography device acquisition document being conducted jointly between the health unit and the supplier involving test actions and adaptation of procedures documented in the health unit so that there is compliance with these applicable technical standards for the equipment, safety instructions issued by the manufacturer and procedures required to ensure the increased equipment working life. During the testing execution phase, the equipment is not available for use with patients until the equipment acceptance certificate is issued jointly by the contract manager, technicians responsible for the use and provider.

Participate in the acceptance testing: (a) the user of equipment; (b) the person responsible for approving the payment of the equipment; (c) the person responsible for managing assets; and (d) the person responsible for equipment operators′ training.

After the acceptance testing phase, trainings are initiated with users and technicians who will operate the mammography device. The equipment supplier shall provide the necessary training to ensure that each service agent is able to perform his/her activities. The training performed aims at individually qualifying each employee involved in the use and availability of equipment, involving even the administrative activities. The training content was been previously discussed between the provider and the health unit, including training regarding security standards in legal and normative acts.

The training sessions provided by the supplier were documented and signed by the participants. The documentation involves from all approached syllabus, attendance record, evaluation of the effectiveness of training and provision for dealing with doubts and questions.

After the training phase, only skilled professionals are allowed to handle the mammography device, implying a greater patient safety. The radiology technician before operating the equipment performs configuration tests and records the values obtained in a proper book in order to ensure traceability procedures. As it is an ionizing radiation emitting equipment, all procedures follow the provisions of the National Council for Nuclear Energy (CNEN).

The mammography device in use at the health unit was purchased less than two years and, therefore, it is covered by the manufacturer′s warranty contract. Thus, the services of preventive and corrective maintenance are scheduled by the equipment supplier, providing a greater equipment availability.

Despite the manufacturer's warranty coverage, the health service has an equipment maintenance policy already documented comprising: (a) the metrological traceability of the equipment; (b) inspections, testing, maintenance, adjustment and calibration of the equipment. All technical interventions made by the equipment supplier are documented in the historical record of the equipment.

The hospital established a systematic approach to preventive and corrective maintenance of the facilities and mammography equipment, being documented on physical media, without a computerized system for recording maintenance actions.

In case of need to perform corrective maintenance procedures, the equipment is then deactivated and the structure required for the maintenance to be performed with the provision of appropriate equipment and tools to do so is installed in the machine room itself. To this end, the health unit maintains a flow of procedures since the perception of an equipment failure by the user until its solution, by the service provider. The systematic approach developed by the health unit encompasses recording failure in a proper form, call record, deadline for implementation of services and reservations regarding the possibility of acquiring pieces in national territory or if imported (which affects the execution time of services).

The space dedicated for use by maintenance staff is sized and compatible with the activities developed, and maintained in good repair, cleaning and hygiene status, protection against the entry of insects and rodents, featuring electrical installations, lighting and air conditioning systems required for health maintenance equipment and the activities performed, according to the manufacturer's recommendation, and it is even possible to track the effect of environmental temperature on the mammography device.

All documents relating to the technical intervention are subsequently attached to the historical documents of the equipment, producing a medical chart where all phases of equipment life cycle are reported.

The person in charge of the health service follows up the interventions and preventive maintenance procedures performed by the provider's technicians based on standard records, aiming to analyze that the actions required to verify that the equipment is in working condition and according to their specifications.

With respect to the mammography device installed at health unit, there are no reports of adverse events related to the equipment. The patients reported some discomfort, resulting from the pressure needed to be done on the breasts during the exam. The administration of the radiology unit considers that this discomfort is common, and there is no need to notify both the manufacturer and the National Health Surveillance System. The procedures for investigating adverse events are described in the unit, should they occur.

The health unit maintains a historical record of mammography equipment, comprising: (a) the identification of the unit at the health facility where the equipment is allocated; (b) professional appointed by the health service responsible for the equipment use; (c) history of equipment failures; (d) documented history of problems and incidents related to adverse events caused, or potentially caused by equipment failures; (e) documentation of technical interventions on the equipment.

Historical records of equipment are filed in the radiology unit itself, under the safeguard of the person responsible for the unit.

Prior to the acquisition of mammography device in use, there was another analog machine installed at the health unit. This machine was donated to another health unit because it was still able to be used. This fact prevented the hospital to be concerned about the disposal of the equipment, so it was enough that the document was transfered to another health facility. Care involved in this phase focused on how to disassemble the equipment in use until then without damaging it and be mounted on the receiving unit to maintain its usability.

It is worth noting that in the health unit analyzed, the mammography equipment is available since its installation, having stopped just in time for the scheduled maintenance. The maximum wait time allowed for completion of a mammogram is seven days after its appointment, and the unit has realistically fulfilled this goal, and so there are no queues for the exam by the target audience of the hospital.

6. Further research

The research performed focused on unraveling the events related to the technology management through clinical engineering. It is extremely important to emphasize that based on the root causes of the problem reported by the TCU report it would still be necessary to consider other aspects that influence the low incidence of mammograms and the consequent early diagnosis of breast cancer in the population.

Accordingly, future studies that can be used throughout the life cycle of the equipment are recommended, involving preliminary technical studies that may indicate in addition to the need of equipment focused on the growing demand for mammograms, the manner to improve their geographic distribution in a country of continental dimensions like Brazil. Technical issues involving the purchase of mammography equipment are coupled with factors such as availability of technical and administrative personnel in a sufficient amount, qualified and motivated.

Studies for expanding the supply of basic inputs such as films and reagents required for their development or installation of equipment that can scan images in order to minimize the need for films, including having an effect on the environment. Moreover, another issue to be analyzed and studied supports the best way to provide information to the public about the importance of the exams within the minimum intervals recommended by the Ministry of Health.

7. Conclusion

Brazil is a country of continental dimensions and problems of the same magnitude. Within the health sector, the problems related to health services management (in all its variations) show that there is a significant gap between what is done by the State to provide health care for the population and their quality expectations.

It is already known by the State that the demographic and epidemiological transitions that the country is subjected to will be reflected across the health system in a few years, because with the aging population, the burden of non-communicable chronic diseases tends to increase, which is different in countries with a predominantly young population.

In terms of the legal and political apparatus existing in the country supporting the creation of health programs, whose purpose is to increase of quality of life for the population, the problems reported by the TCU in relation to the low productivity of mammograms are presented only as a small link in a chain of problems.

Most of these problems approached in the report, are associated with the absence of prior planning for the purchase and installation of mammography equipment. Notwithstanding this fact, the case study revealed that it is possible to reach a condition of increased availability of mammography equipment, with the participation of the Clinical Engineering as part of the decision making and management processes.

In a process of analysis and correction of problems, the Clinical Engineering within its competence scope, would act on the equipment management, providing both the planning of the necessary infrastructure and the equipment support after its purchase. The direct and indirect benefits of the action of the Clinical engineering can be seen through increased safety for patients and technical staff because, as processes and procedures for maintenance of mammography devices, as well as their periodic calibrations and measurements are there was a direct reflection on the nonoccurrence of adverse events arising from the use of mammography device.

Another relevant aspect is the fact that the increased availability of mammography devices, has direct effects on the economy of the health facility, because the presence of a non-effective equipment imposes upon this facility the cost of obsolescence and technological gap without the provision of its direct purpose, namely, the ability to provide early breast cancer diagnosis. The possibility of the occurrence of this condition is even more serious, whereas the facility would have means of diagnosing it early if the equipment was not out of operation.

Regarding the application of standardized procedures by ABNT NBR 15943: 2011, their effects are measured directly on the availability of mammography devices, since the standard is concerned to provide important steps to be followed throughout the organization, taking care of the equipment life cycle from the planning phase of its acquisition to its final disposal.

During the research at the health care facility, we observed the attention given by professionals to meet the guidelines set forth in the standard from the initial conception of the acquisition of the mammography device, disabling of the equipment that was in use, the new equipment installation, analysis, issuing of reports and testing, technical staff training, provision of maintenance and support by the clinical engineering. All these factors were reflected in the availability of the equipment in full time, considering the low waiting time on the part of the target audience to achieve the performance of a mammogram.

Nomenclature

Competent sanitary authority: an authority who is responsible, in his/her territorial demarcation, for the implementation of appropriate sanitary measures in accordance with the laws and regulations prevailing in the national territory, international treaties and other acts, of which Brazil is a signatory.

Calibration: a set of operations that establish, under specified conditions, the relationship between values indicated by a measuring instrument or measuring system, values represented by a material measure or a reference material and the corresponding values of the quantities set forth by standards.

Availability: capacity of an item to be able to perform a certain function at a given time or during a given time interval, taking into account the combined aspects of its reliability, maintainability and maintenance support, assuming that the required external resources are ensured.

Health equipment: a set of devices and machines, parts and accessories used by a health care setting where diagnosis actions, therapy and monitoring are developed. Shall be considered health equipment those support, infrastructure, and general medical care devices.

Medical-care equipment: equipment or system, including their accessories and parts, of usage or medical, dental or laboratory application, used directly or indirectly for diagnosis, therapy and monitoring in health care of the population, and which do not use pharmacological, immunological or metabolic means to perform their main function in humans, whereas being able to be assisted in their functions by such means.

Adverse events: damage to health caused to a patient or user due to the use of a product subject to sanitary surveillance regime, whereas its use is carried out under conditions and parameters prescribed by the manufacturer.

Health technology management: a set of management procedures planned and implemented from scientific and technical, normative and legal bases in order to ensure traceability, quality, efficacy, effectiveness, safety and in some cases the performance of health technologies used in the provision of health services. It covers every step of management, from planning and admission into the health unit until its disposal, in order to protect workers, the preservation of public health and the environment and patient safety.

Maintenance: a combination of all technical and administrative actions, including supervisionto maintain or replace an item in a state in which it can perform a required function.

Management Plan: a document indicating and describing the criteria established by the health facility for performing the management steps of different health technologies subject to health inspection and supervision from planning and admission into the health care setting, until its use in health and disposal services.

Traceability: the capacity to trace the history, application or location of an item by means of previously recorded information.

http://dx.doi.org/10.5772/60792

Acknowledgements

Special thanks to the Laboratory of Health Informatics (LIS) at the University of Brasília, at Gama (FGA), for providing an important space for learning and information exchange between teachers and students. Thanks are intended for professionals in the health care unit who welcomed us carefully and dedicated their precious time to provide the requested information.

Author details

Cleber da Silva Alves*, Marília Miranda Forte Gomes and Lourdes Mattos Brasil

*Address all correspondence to: alves-cleber@hotmail.com

Post Graduate Program in Biomedical Engineering at the University of Brasília (UnB) at Gama (FGA), Brazil

References

[1] Brasil. Constituição. Constituição da República Federativa do Brasil. Brasília, DF, Senado; 1988.

[2] Brasil. Lei 8080 de 19 de setembro de 1990. http://www.planalto.gov.br/ccivil_03/leis/l8080.htm. (accessed 08 November 2014).

[3] Rede Interagencial de Informações Para Saúde. Informe de situação e tendências: demografia e saúde / Rede Interagencial de Informações para Saúde. – Brasília: Organização Pan-Americana da Saúde; 2009. 36 p. : il. – (Série G. Estatística e Informação em Saúde) (Série Informe de Situação e Tendências)

[4] Malta Dc et al. Epidemiologia das doenças crônicas não transmissíveis no Brasil. In ROUQUAYROL MZ & SILVA MGC (ed). Epidemiologia & Saúde. 7. ed. Rio de Janeiro: MedBook; 2013.

[5] Duncan Bb et al. Mortalidade por doencas cronicas no Brasil: situacão em 2009 e tendencias de 1991 a 2009. In. In Saúde Brasil 2010: uma análise da situacão de saúde e de evidencias selecionadas de impacto de acões de vigilancia em saúde. Ministério da Saúde, Secretaria de Vigilancia em Saúde, Departamento de Análise de Situacão em Saúde: Brasilia; 2011.

[6] WHO. Breast cancer: prevention and control. World Health Organization. http://www.who.int/cancer/detection/breastcancer/en (accessed 03 May 2014).

[7] Brasil. Ministério da Saúde. Secretaria de Vigilância em Saúde. Departamento de Análise de Situação de Saúde. Saúde Brasil 2011 : uma análise da situação de saúde e

a vigilância da saúde da mulher / Ministério da Saúde, Secretaria de Vigilância em Saúde, Departamento de Análise de Situação de Saúde. – Brasília : Editora do Ministério da Saúde; 2012. 444 p. : il.

[8] Inca. Ministério da Saúde. Estimativa 2014: Incidencia de Câncer no Brasil / Instituto Nacional de Câncer José Alencar Gomes da Silva, Coordenacão de Prevenção e Vigilância. Rio de Janeiro: INCA; 2014.

[9] Inca. Ministério da Saúde. Controle do câncer de mama: documento de consenso. Rio de Janeiro: INCA; 2004.

[10] Inca. Ministério da Saúde. Parâmetros Técnicos para Programação de Ações de Detecção Precoce do Câncer de Mama: recomendações para gestores estaduais e municipais. Rio de Janeiro: INCA; 2006.

[11] Lima-Costa Mf, Matos Dl. Prevalência e fatores associados à realização da mamografia na faixa etária de 50-69 anos: um estudo baseado na Pesquisa Nacional por Amostra de Domicílios (2003). Cad. Saúde Pública [online]; 2007. vol.23, n.7, pp. 1665-1673.

[12] Pinotti Ja, Pinotti M. Prevenção do Câncer de Mama. Em Antunes RCP, Perdicaris AAM, editores. Prevenção do Câncer. Barueri: Manole; 2010. p. 237.

[13] Tcu Acórdão No 247/2010 – Tcu – Plenário.

[14] Brasil. Conselho Nacional de Secretários de Saúde. Ciência e Tecnologia em Saúde / Conselho Nacional de Secretários de Saúde. – Brasília : CONASS; 2007.

[15] Calil, SJ. Gerenciamento de Manutencão de Equipamentos Hospitalares, volume 11. São Paulo: Faculdade de Saúde Pública da Universidade de São Paulo; 1998.

[16] ACCE Definition. American College of Clinical engineering. http://www.accenet.org/default.asp?page=about&section=definition (accessed 04 November 2014).

[17] Brasil. Ministério da Saúde. Instituto Nacional do Câncer. e-SIC Sistema Eletrônico do Serviço de Informação ao Cidadão. Protocolo 25820003703201471. http://www.acessoainformacao.gov.br/sistema/site/index.html (accessed 04 November 2014).

[18] Associação Brasileira De Normas Técnicas. Nbr 15943. Diretrizes para um programa de gerenciamento de equipamentos de infraestrutura de serviços de saúde e de equipamentos para a saúde. Rio de Janeiro; 2011.

[19] Shi L. Health services research methods. 2. ed. New York: Delmar Cengage Learning; 2008.

[20] Yin, Rk. Estudo de caso: planejamento e métodos. Tradução Daniel Grassi. 3. ed. Porto Alegre: Bookman; 2005.

http://dx.doi.org/10.5772/60792

[21] Brasil. Agência Nacional de Vigilância Sanitária. RDC 2, de 25 de janeiro de 2010. Dispõe sobre o gerenciamento de tecnologias em saúde em estabelecimentos de saúde. Brasília; 2010.

[22] Brasil. Lei 8.666 de 21 de junho de 1993. http://www.planalto.gov.br/ccivil 03/leis/l8666cons.htm (accessed 08 November 2014).